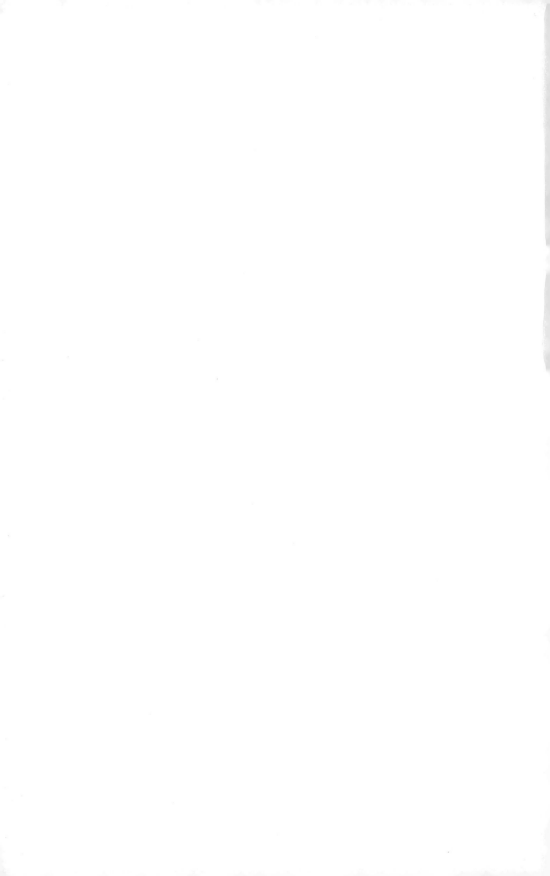

The Healthy Home

The
Healthy Home

Simple Truths to Protect Your Family
From Hidden Household Dangers

Dave Wentz and Dr. Myron Wentz
with Donna K. Wallace

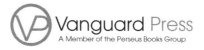
Vanguard Press
A Member of the Perseus Books Group

Designed by Nathan Parét
Set in 11 point Adobe Garmond Pro and 9 point Gill Sans

Cataloging-in-Publication data for this book is available from the Library
of Congress.
ISBN 13: 978-1-59315-655-8

Vanguard Press books are available at special discounts for bulk purchases in the
U.S. by corporations, institutions, and other organizations. For more information,
please contact the Special Markets Department at the Perseus Books Group, 2300
Chestnut Street, Suite 200, Philadelphia, PA 19103, or call (800) 810-4145,
ext. 5000, or e-mail special.markets@perseusbooks.com.

10 9 8 7 6 5 4 3 2 1

To Andrew, our reason for finally committing these words to paper. You make us feel hopeful for the future.

Author Note

Dave Wentz and Dr. Myron Wentz will donate 100 percent of their proceeds

from sales of *The Healthy Home* to effective nonprofit organizations that

help nourish, educate, and provide medical care for impoverished children.

Leading this group of notable charitable organizations is Children's Hunger

Fund (CHF), with which the authors have partnered for many years.

Please visit www.myhealthyhome.com/charity for more information on how

you can help.

Contents

WELCOME   1

Contents

The Healthy Home

Introduction

Over the years I've rarely had to ask my dad, Dr. Myron Wentz, what he thinks about major issues of the day.

All I had to do was observe what he was actually doing—both with his time and the financial means he had at his disposal. Improvements in diagnostic medicine, development of quality nutritional supplements, research in holistic medicine, aid for malnourished orphans, support for the fine arts—his passions are many, but his methods rarely change.

He's taught me that tangible, personal actions are what make a real difference.

And if individual efforts aren't enough to bring about desired change, he would say, "Well, you could always write a book."

I found myself thinking about my dad's example in recent years as I prepared for and welcomed the birth of my first child. Suddenly I faced a new and sobering responsibility—to keep Andrew safe from harm. For a long time one of my constant concerns has been our unnecessary exposure to hidden environmental toxins in daily life. Every second of every day, we face an onslaught of unnecessary dangers—toxic chemicals, negative energies, unforeseen side effects, and more—in our modern world.

With Andrew's impending arrival, my concern for these hidden dangers grew into a true passion. And as I'd learned from my father, passion means action.

As much as I would have liked to do so, there was no way to take on every toxic manufacturer or sluggish government regulator. But I did know of something I could do that would make a huge difference for Andrew and many others. It was best explained through two simple words—awareness and avoidance. By enhancing our knowledge about environmental health hazards and lessening our exposure to such risks, I was certain I could help others improve their chances for long-term health and ensure the future well-being of their children.

Because of Andrew, I wanted to tell the people around me about the dangers lurking in things they take for granted every day. I wanted to explain how to remove—or at least lessen—those dangers in the home, easily and without great inconvenience. I wanted to offer hope that even small changes, when added up over many years, could make an incredible difference. It was time to take my father's advice—and write a book.

So I called in the experts.

First, my dad, whose vast knowledge and voracious appetite for research have allowed him to see between the lines of studies and speculation. Second, Donna K. Wallace, a writer who has co-authored several notable health books and has made a career out of helping busy executives like me look better in print.

Together, we set out to prove that you don't have to be a scientist—or even a cave-dwelling technophobe—to protect your family from the toxic influences found in modern society. You don't have to accept products or habits that are dangerous. The following pages will show you how you can make a difference.

You can have a healthy home.

The first step is learning. The second step is taking decisive action to change your life. That part will be up to you.

—Dave Wentz

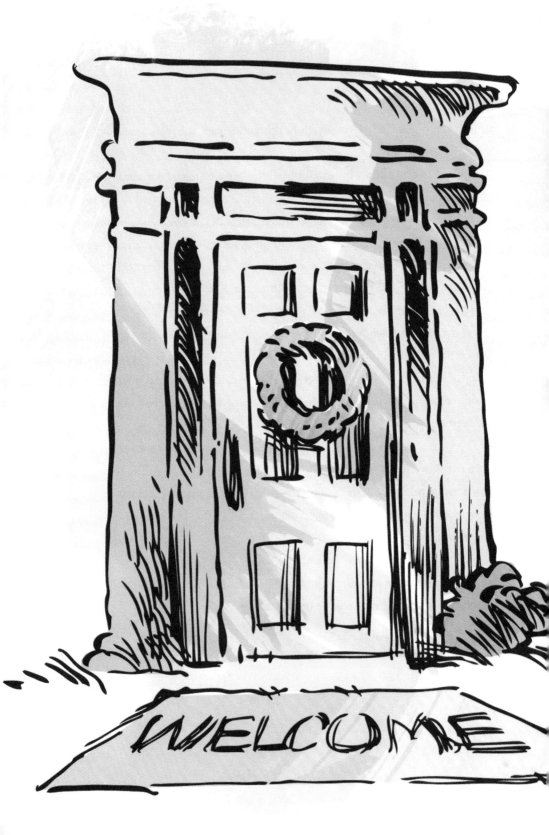

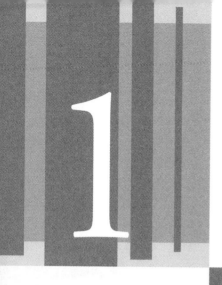

1

Welcome

by Donna K. Wallace

Salt Lake City is home to Dave Wentz, recently named by Forbes.com as "One of America's Most Powerful CEOs 40 and Under." Dave has accomplished much within his first four decades, including helping his father, Dr. Myron Wentz, found USANA Health Sciences, the international nutritional company that Dave now leads. I'm excited to discover what he has in mind for the project that brought me here.

I arrive at an impressive glass building that reflects budding trees, beautiful xeriscaping, and the drama of the city's signature mountain ranges. I am then escorted to Dave's office, a grand corner affair with spectacular views. A treadmill occupies a prominent position near the neatly organized desk.

Dave stands and greets me with a polite hug. Fit and tan, his skin shows little sign of aging. He's doing something right. Shy, but with a focus that burns through any possible inhibitions, his personal, casual demeanor quickly puts me at ease.

We chat briefly, then he stands again and gestures for me to follow him back through the door.

Dave walks with me to the company's "Creative Room," a bright space with a hodgepodge of beanbag chairs, ottomans, and armchairs. White markerboards wrap entirely around the room, some still exhibiting the remnants of earlier brainstorming sessions. An assistant brings us nutritious snacks: health bars, mixed nuts and fruit, water, and the company's healthy energy drink that is served in lieu of coffee.

Once we're settled, Dave gets right down to it.

Dave: To tell the truth, I'm pretty far out of my comfort zone in writing a book, but there's a serious need for this one to be written, so that's why you're here. I need you to help me organize the information I have and help me express it in a way that will reach out to the people who need it.

Donna: What motivated you to undertake such a huge project?

Dave: The hidden dangers of everyday things we consume or that surround us—things that have a direct impact on our health. Yet our governing agencies don't have the time or means to regulate them, medical professionals choose to ignore them until they reveal themselves as physical symptoms, and regular people don't even realize they're an issue.

We need to get folks talking about these things. It's only then that we can enable people to avoid these dangers or, at the very least, be aware of their impact.

Donna: Are there specific things you want to address over the course of the project?

Dave: It's difficult knowing where to begin, and that's part of why you're here—we need to organize this into something people can really use. Just off the top of my head I can name *[ticking off each item as he identifies it]* . . .

- That "new car smell" is so dangerous it ought to deploy an airbag.
- Those silver fillings in your mouth could one day prevent you from recognizing your own reflection.
- Your microwave isn't a television, so by all means *don't* watch your popcorn pop.
- If you wouldn't drink it, don't put it on your skin.
- Your scented laundry acts like a nicotine patch.
- We poison our homes just to kill a fly.
- Plastic may steal your family's future.
- We don't really know the long-term consequences of vaccinations.
- Indoor air pollution is the asbestos of tomorrow.
- Technological advancements made for profit will always outpace research designed for safety.
- Fluoride is poisonous.
- You have to be careful whose advice you buy.
- You are your own best advocate.
- Moderation—not abstinence—is usually the solution to excess.

And that's just the beginning.

Donna: That's quite a beginning, yet this seems like a strange project for a CEO, even if you do run a health sciences company. What motivates you—and *qualifies* you—to undertake such a mission?

Dave: It really stems from my father's scientific research. My dad, Dr. Myron Wentz, is one of the world's leading authorities on cellular nutrition. He received the Albert Einstein Award for Achievement in the Life Sciences and has always been relentless in his pursuit of health breakthroughs.

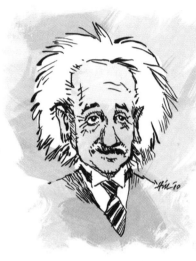

Because of my unique upbringing and my experience helping found a health-focused company with my father, I'm surrounded by truths that I assumed most people knew already. But the deeper I dig, the more I've learned that the vast majority of people remain blissfully—and dangerously—unaware.

Donna: Does your father share your opinions?

Dave: Very much so. His belief is that, due to the onslaught of toxins in the environment, coupled with poor nutrition and unhealthy lifestyles, our children may be the first generation of kids that may not live as long as their parents. I mean, the evidence isn't hard to find. It's all around us. For this very reason, I didn't want to have children of my own—I didn't want them to suffer in a toxic world that we created. But over time that changed, and now I have a young son of my own.

When my wife, Reneé, was pregnant, I couldn't sleep at night, hoping that she was getting the nutrition she needed and worrying about the toxins she might have been exposed to—that day and in the past. As I'd feel the baby kick or roll, I was filled with wonder, but I also worried about our child's future.

Now our son, Andrew, is exploring a bigger world. Now that he's out of the womb, we have far less control over the things that affect him in profound and frightening ways. This has led me to question more than ever before.

Is it even possible to make a big enough difference in the world to redirect the current trends? Or will we be battling a new evolutionary challenge of man-made toxins, in which degenerative diseases like cancer, heart disease, and Alzheimer's are the norm? I hope we can make the change for *his* future. Regardless of what the world does, I'm going to empower myself to give him the best opportunity for a healthy, happy life.

Andrew will be healthy by choice, not by chance.

Donna: With such an important mission as "protecting your family," will it be possible to break it down into manageable steps?

Dave: I believe it can, or we wouldn't be having this conversation. To begin with, I'd recommend that people do four basic things:

- **Count the cost of convenience.** Decide what you can't live without and reassess the rest, because convenience can kill.
- **Live by the Precautionary Principle**—"It's better to be safe than sorry." In the process, listen to your instincts. Don't assume that because something's common it's safe.
- **Let your senses be your guide.** In this toxic world, the nose knows.
- And although the government may choose economy over ecology, **do the opposite.** Health is more important than money. Don't wait for others to protect your family—do it yourself, starting in your own home.

We can't let it become overwhelming. Once we learn the truth, it's easy to become despondent about the onslaught of toxins bombarding our bodies each day. Our readers must understand that they don't have to accomplish *everything* we recommend in this book. Adopting even one good habit will make a person healthier; several positive changes can improve a person's quality of life; and with each added step, our readers can extend their lives—and the lives of their family members—by years.

Knowing what I do, I'm filled with hope for my son's generation. We are learning how to be aware—how to be our own best advocates. Parents are getting involved in ensuring their families' safety. Our children are fortunate to follow in the footsteps of visionaries like my father.

My son Andrew is the grandchild of a man who has impacted hundreds of thousands of lives. When you go to the doctor's office to have your blood drawn— perhaps to test for a viral infection such as mononucleosis—the lab will likely be using diagnostic technology my father developed many years ago. He could have stopped there, but when he realized that diagnosing disease didn't reach far enough, he went back to cellular technology to discover ways to combat degenerative diseases and identify the means for prevention.

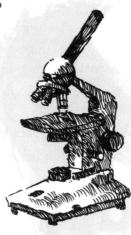

We still have a long way to go, but so often I see people taking notice and making choices to live well and live long. That's why this book is needed. I'm not the only one raising a child in this world.

Donna: With so much information at our fingertips, doesn't everyone already have the knowledge they need to keep themselves safe?

Dave: History has taught us that, with most major discoveries and for many exciting new products, there's a lengthy gap in time before product safety information travels from the lab to the public. In most cases, it takes too long to measure conclusive evidence. By the time a product may be determined to be unsafe, lives almost certainly will have been lost.

This is where the Precautionary Principle comes in. The principle states that when an activity or product has the potential of causing harm to human health or the environment, precautionary measures should be taken, even if the cause-and-effect relationship hasn't been completely established through the scientific process.

Science can't go fast enough. We *must* rely on personal logic and intuition until science gets there. Each one of us must take in all the information available—along with a large measure of common sense and a willingness to forego convenience and the latest innovations. We must reawaken our senses to those things we know or believe to be true.

Donna: Given that your father is a scientist, how do you reconcile the fact that you're putting intuition before science?

Dave: It's not so contradictory as you might suspect.

Growing up, I had as a father the scientist who came with giant unpronounceable words, unleashed complicated descriptions of the simplest things, and expressed endless opinions on every action and reaction we encountered in our daily lives. I remember as a kid playing with my friends in the dirt and a neighbor warning us not to put the dirt in our mouths. My dad heard and replied, "Let them eat the dirt. It will build their immune systems."

So many times we do things—or don't do things—without stopping to ask "why?" My dad uses his intuition to ask "why" to nearly everything.

The important thing was that he always had an endless desire to learn, which took him to scientific meetings all over the world, frequently taking me with him. At fourteen, I learned that the Germans were very much into detoxing by sweating in a sauna and then rolling in the snow or taking a plunge into icy water. I was shocked and fascinated by this, not because of the health benefits I was learning but because they did it in the nude . . . and it was co-ed.

That was an eye-opener: One culture's norm is another's taboo.

There were some really cool aspects to being the son of a mad scientist who had his sights set on bringing widespread change. But I sometimes wished I had a dad who would come home, kick his shoes off, watch a movie with me . . . I don't know, maybe shoot hoops in the driveway or something. But my father has always had a one-track mind. Even though he has a broad perspective and many different interests, he has one driving passion. He approaches everything from the viewpoint of a scientist, 24/7.

It can be maddening. My father's global vision of "true health" never wanes. He is on a tireless pursuit of his Holy Grail—the next breakthrough to ease the world's suffering and disease.

Donna: But doesn't that lead to the perspective of a person whose theories only exist on paper?

Dave: Not at all. My father has been a student his whole life. He never stops studying and learning, and he sees things most people don't. What seems intuitive to us is mere logic to him. For him, life isn't about rushing through each day and getting everything done on our to-do list. Life is about living.

In fact, his work extends far beyond the laboratory. He's very focused on building hospitals in third world countries and often travels with the international charity Children's Hunger Fund. All of our proceeds from this book will help support CHF and other charities like it.

CHILDREN'S HUNGER FUND

As an example of his approach, we know that eating greasy, deep-fried fast food isn't the smartest idea. Yet my father made sure that I witnessed for myself—through the microscope—cells actually dying as a result of exposure to things we consume all the time. Those images don't leave much room for debate on what are questionable decisions.

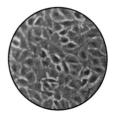

Needless to say, as much as I like burgers and fries, moderation is the rule. I temper my desire to really indulge myself with the knowledge that I'll be sacrificing a lot of happy, healthy cells. I'm not perfect, but I'm definitely healthier because I'm aware.

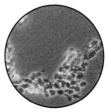

So along the way I've learned to see and understand the world in much the same way as my father does. He speaks a language that only a small number of highly specialized people can understand. I'm technically educated in bioengineering, but I suppose I learned most of what I know by osmosis. I'm sort of like an immigrant's child who must learn to communicate on a parent's behalf after moving to a new country; my life has centered on explaining what my dad means and doing so in layman's terms.

I am my father's translator to the world. He understands what true health looks like through the microscope, and I explain it simply enough for most to understand.

Donna: Nevertheless, his knowledge sounds highly specialized. Can you explain this in a way that can be grasped and implemented by everyone who reads the book?

Dave: I know I can. I have the foundation of my father's accomplishments, but I actually despise long, dusty lectures on scientific findings. I'm easily distracted; I want to provide quick answers and practical solutions. I want people to succeed at moderation rather than fail at absolute abstinence—to know about small changes that can be made easily, and will have a lifetime of impact.

My business takes me around the world, so I see endless global needs. But this book will allow us to focus closer to home. I don't know about you, but when I get to choose, I want to be home with my family. Yes, the world matters, and we all need to do our part, but I can see it starting at home in my living room.

And it can be that way for everyone. I'm not trying to write a comprehensive rulebook for danger-proofing one's life. Changing an entire lifestyle is way too arduous for *anyone*, especially when people are so busy that convenience seems the only way to go. No, we need to make people aware of dangers they didn't know about or hadn't really thought about, offer readers simple solutions that they can actually implement and not even notice or mind, and help people live healthier lives.

We can do that for families everywhere.

Donna: Hamburgers aside, though, can readers expect to live the ideal lifestyle you must have led in a household like yours?

Dave: With a father like mine, it could be assumed that I grew up in some sort of vegan, technology-free, sterile environment.

But the truth is that I didn't.

My dad by no means knows it all, but his advantage is that he doesn't let ignorance become an excuse to stick to the norm and not rock the boat. If he suspects there's a hidden issue—on anything from bottled water to tattoo ink—he researches it until he uncovers an answer. Sometimes it's not the answer he expected. Scientific theory is based on the premise that each new theory will either be disproven or expanded.

A true scientist never speaks emphatically, as if he or she has the final answer.

My father has definitely switched opinions on various issues as he's gathered more information, but the important thing is that he's still ahead of the curve.

To this day I harass him for feeding me Vienna sausages on camping trips when I was a kid. Now, after years of studying health and prevention, the thought that he actually fed me processed pork and chicken canned in a salty, preservative-laden jelly is appalling to him. He didn't think about the ramifications then, but he certainly does now. He's *constantly* learning, so that in the future, when he looks back, there will be fewer instances he will want to kick himself for. I consider that the model I took away from my upbringing.

And we're not creating fire here. After searching through everything from volumes of scholarly journals to goofy marketing scams, I want to provide a simple, trustworthy guide. I want our readers to get maximum information in a format that's quick and easy to read with tons of solutions—a whole range of them that will fit any budget. You can make a handful of changes that will have a cumulative effect over a lifetime and may alter the course of your life.

No agenda or mind-numbing statistics—just the freedom to make your own choices. It's about learning what's out there and realizing the ability to maximize your choices. There are many ways to live well. But health always comes back to the cell. When our cells are healthy, we're healthy.

Donna: "Go Green" is very fashionable right now. Will the recommendations in this book work within that philosophy, and if so, how?

Dave: Living green is on everyone's minds. My company has made some major strides in lessening our environmental impact and reducing our waste, and that's important for all of us to do. But this isn't about the environment out there; the environment's right here, surrounding us all the time. Our most important ecosystems are our homes and workplaces. They're either making us well or making us sick. Each of us is a cellular being who interacts with every substance we encounter no matter how miniscule it is. What we're after here is true health—making the space in which we live as safe as it's meant to be.

If we can accomplish this, we're golden.

Donna: But there will need to be a model for the reader to follow—an example that will give form to the ideas you want to communicate.

Dave: Well, I think I have just the thing. Reneé and I are just finishing a massive remodel and we're just getting the house back together. The whole, crazy process has probably taken months out of my life—but it probably added years, in the balance. We intentionally got rid of some things, such as old carpet. Instead, we went with easier-to-clean tile and hardwood floors with nontoxic glues and finishes. We made sure to include air cleaners and water filters. We're making small, gradual changes that will have long-term effects.

That seems like the ideal place to begin . . .

■ ■ ■

A Healthy Home Tour

Dave insisted that we explore real solutions—for example, what each of us could do in about fifteen minutes that would make a difference. In his life, he said, he'd roll up his sleeves—armed with a trash bag and shovel, if need be—in order to bring about change. The simple truths, he added, lie in knowing *why* we need to take action, and then making it happen.

So what hits closest to home?

Home.

Your house may be a temporary hangout or a "step home." It might be an apartment or your dream home. Whether you plan to reside there for three years or thirty, home is the environment in which you eat, sleep, work, and play—ultimately the backdrop for good health or disease. This book is framed in the blueprint of a house that will also become a blueprint for living better, safer, healthier lives—step by step, room by room.

One of Dr. Myron Wentz's most famous quotes is this:

"We live too short and die too long."

He's made it his life's work to change that. A visionary in cellular science, he believes that to live fully means lowering the risk for all disease and maximizing health at the cellular level. So many choices we make and things we encounter every day of our lives will impact our ability to live fully until we die. These include what we choose to eat and drink, where we sleep, what we put on our skin, and how we clean our homes.

We've heard more than our fair share about living in a "toxic soup." Scientific studies can be discouraging, and we can become desensitized to hearing that there's danger at every turn.

This book isn't a litany of environmental dangers, with lengthy and depressing lists of chemicals and toxins. Instead, it will concentrate on a select few of Dave's and Dr. Wentz's greatest concerns—many of which may surprise you—that they chose to focus on in their own homes. This fits with Dave's mission to make a difference and provide a range of simple solutions to minimize your risk while creating a healthier environment where your family can thrive.

The Tools of the Trade

If we're honest, convenience and budget have a lot to do with determining what changes we choose to make. In addition to the book's essential facts and quick, cost-effective action steps, Dr. Wentz will provide deeper science for those who want it. After exposing shocking truths and the science that unlocks the mystery behind them, we'll put into perspective the dangers you'll see and the choices you'll make in the days, weeks, months, and years to come.

Each section will focus on a specific part of the home, revealing surprising ramifications for your health while providing insight into the inner workings and unknown effects on your body. With a quick flip through the pages you'll find:

- cartoons that provide quick visuals for important information;
- quizzes at the beginning of each chapter enabling you to measure your current lifestyle and better choose which solutions are appropriate for you;
- "Cellular Truths" boxes from Dr. Wentz that offer descriptions of what is happening on a fundamental level as well as less formal "Ask the Scientist" boxes that highlight his personal responses to a range of questions;
- health risks associated with specific dangers and antidotes designed to combat those dangers;
- a range of other solutions—from simple fixes to dramatic changes; and
- links to the book's Web site, which will offer more detailed information and help you create a personalized plan for creating a healthier home.

Dave Wentz will walk us through each page, translating and prioritizing our greatest challenges while his father—always in hot pursuit of the truth—will examine them with a kind of x-ray vision, the result of having peered through a microscope for so many years and uncovering what lay there.

To get a broader spectrum of the science behind this book, please visit www.myhealthyhome.com.

The Tour Begins

The next day Dave is waiting at the front door of his home, a stylish second-story loft that's part of a converted warehouse in historic downtown Salt Lake City. His father, Dr. Myron Wentz, arrives soon after, carrying with him a small bag. A visionary who has dedicated his life to creating innovative solutions to the world's health problems, Dr. Wentz shares his son's passion for making the home a safe, nontoxic place. And conversation with Dave and Dr. Wentz comes packaged with its own rhythm of science and humor.

Dave: This feels a little awkward, but I think we need to start in the bedroom because this is where we spend the majority of our time in the home—humanity, I mean.

Dr. Wentz: I imagine it is also where life begins for most of us.

He tosses Dave a glance, and the three of us walk down a corridor where we are greeted by the sounds of a waterfall. The first thing to hit me is how clean Dave's home smells—as though there's really no smell at all.

This is where Dave and Dr. Wentz begin to open our eyes.

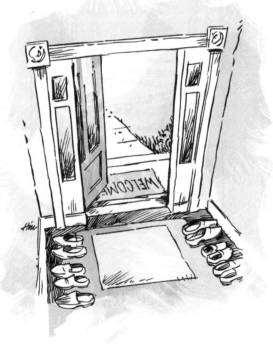

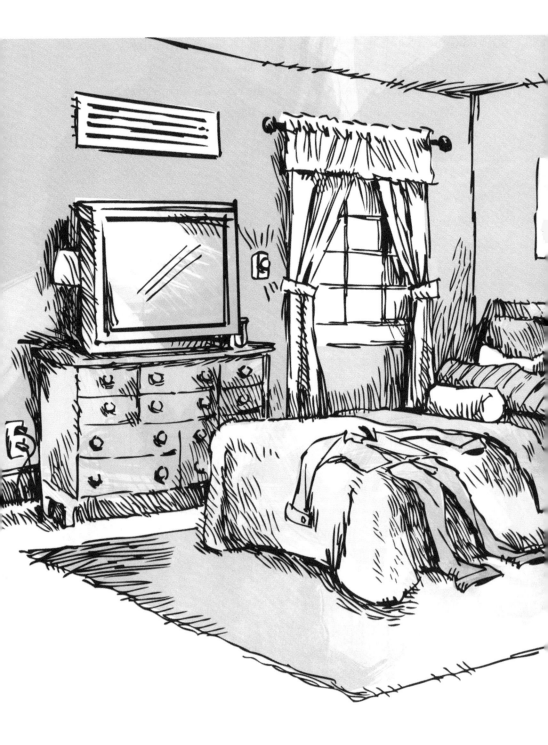

2

The Bedroom

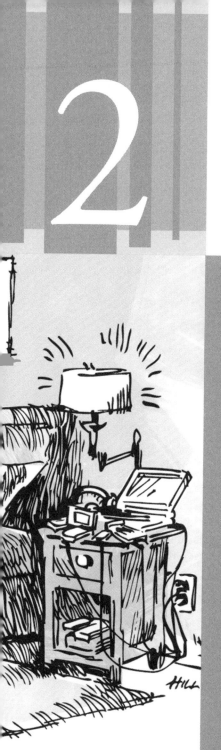

The bedroom—often the crown glory of the home—promises a relaxing and luxurious retreat. Research shows, however, that when it comes to deep and restful sleep, our bedrooms aren't measuring up. For many of us, our most personal room in the house needs a serious makeover, one with solutions that reach beyond designer paint or the latest furniture.

The bedroom plays host to any number of activities, from TV watching to treadmill time. We easily spend at least one-third of our lives there, and our vitality begins there. Without noticing, however, we've allowed dangers to intrude that could be siphoning life rather than replenishing it.

Our own actions may be first in the lineup of suspects.

Some surprisingly simple changes to your bedroom may improve the quality of your sleep and your vitality. Whether you prefer austere or elaborate, sexy chic or cottage comfy, the first room in your home to clean up and clear out is your bedroom. With a few basic insights and some simple solutions, you can make yours a refuge of healthy rejuvenation.

We walk down a hallway past large modern paintings to Dave's bedroom, a room that is simply decorated while exuding classic elegance. A fresh breeze stirs thick drapes that frame a wall of windows looking over downtown Salt Lake City and the Wasatch mountain range to the east. The late morning sun bathes the room in gold-specked light.

Dr. Wentz walks into the middle of his son's newly renovated bedroom, turns 360 degrees, and then takes a big sniff of the duvet before digging under the sheets to look at the label on the mattress.

Donna: What's he doing?

Dave: He's checking to see what chemicals he can smell. Indoor air pollution is one of the top health risks today. It's due to the fact that so many synthetic substances are now used in the construction of our homes, and there are so many toxins in the products we employ. Combined with the lack of air circulation in many homes, indoor air is usually much more polluted than outdoor air.

There's a lot you can do to choose products that carry a lower chemical burden than the usual stuff you find in the stores.

Dr. Wentz: What are all those gadgets on your nightstand?

Dave: I know, I know—at least *some* of them are temporary, like the baby monitor. But, you're right—I need to get the rest out of here.
[*Dr. Wentz walks over to inspect the blinds that hang over the windows.*]

Dr. Wentz: You used to get too much light from that street lamp. Are these new drapes doing the trick?

Dave: Yes, but I doubt I'd notice the light these days. Reneé and I are just too exhausted when we go to bed.

Dr. Wentz: With a baby in the house, I'll bet you are, but there's more to quality sleep than being passed out on the bed. Your hormone balance, which controls proper cellular function and repair at night, is driven by melatonin. Melatonin is produced when it gets dark, and its production can shut off with just a flash of light.

How many times is Andrew getting up each night?

Dave: It's getting better now, but for a while there it was four to five times each night. He has a schedule of his own.

Dr. Wentz: Yes, young children and their different sleep patterns can present a challenge, but I hope you're keeping the lights very low when you tend to him. Even before Andrew was born, it seemed like you kids were competing to see who could get by on the least amount of sleep.

Dave: I know some people who only need five hours of sleep, so I feel like I should be able to get by with the same.

Dr. Wentz: We've always heard that eight hours of sleep each night is a necessity for rebuilding cells, but did you know that too little or too much sleep shortens life? Each person's body is different, so adults need to figure out what is the optimal amount of sleep for them individually.

Donna: So sleep isn't necessarily a "one size fits all" formula, as we've been taught?

Dr. Wentz: Not really, no. Your body has an internal "clock"—a small group of cells located in your brain and known as the suprachiasmatic nucleus. This clock is set by the level of light your eye receives, and it establishes your body's natural sleep-wake rhythm. When the sun begins dipping below the horizon, your body naturally begins winding down for the day.

Donna: The heart beats more slowly, blood pressure lowers, muscles relax . . .

Dr. Wentz: Exactly. One of the functions of our internal clock is to prevent our bodies' systems from disturbing our rest. For example, kidney function drops at night so you don't have to get up several times during the night to relieve yourself. Your body temperature also typically drops. However, getting healthy sleep also depends on *consciously* avoiding not-so-good nighttime activities, such as exercising and eating.

Dave: *[Laughs]* I wish we could tell Andrew that.

Dr. Wentz: Wouldn't that be nice? Fortunately for you and Reneé, sleep quality is just as important as sleep quantity. I believe achieving truly restful sleep is the area where most of us should focus our efforts.

Chapter 1
There's the Rub

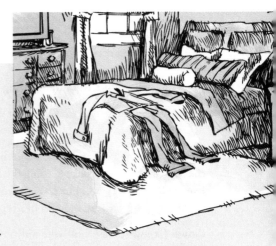

Take a look around your bedroom and you'll see fabric everywhere. From your mattress to your bedding to your closet full of clothing, the bedroom contains a wide array of natural and synthetic fabrics, many of which touch your body for an extended time in a very intimate way.

That new comforter, favorite shirt, or expensive lingerie could be exposing your body to unknown toxins and hidden dangers. It's time to give bedroom fabrics a good once-over.

Quizzes at the beginning of each chapter will help you assess hidden dangers in your home. A higher score signals that you may have a higher risk in a particular area. Save your chapter quiz scores until the end of each room section, where you'll be provided a long list of solutions to even up your score.

QUIZ How Toxic Is Your Home?   Scores

1. Which of the following best describes your bedding and pajamas fabric?
   - [ ] Organic cotton (0 pts)
   - [ ] Synthetic and natural blend (6 pts)
   - [ ] 100 percent natural fabrics like silk, hemp, cotton, wool, etc. (1 pt)
   - [ ] 100 percent synthetics (12 pts)

2. Which products do you typically use for laundry? (Select all that apply)
   - [ ] Scented detergent (6 pts)
   - [ ] Dryer sheets (6 pts)
   - [ ] Stain treatments (3 pts)
   - [ ] Fabric softener (6 pts)
   - [ ] Static cling spray (3 pts)
   - [ ] Fragrance-free detergent (0 pts)

3. Which of the following clothing and accessory items leave red lines on your skin? (Select all that apply)
   - [ ] Undergarments (8 pts)
   - [ ] Collar/Tie (6 pts)
   - [ ] Belt/Pants waistband (8 pts)
   - [ ] Socks (3 pts) [ ] Jewelry/Watches (3 pts)

4. How many days a week do you typically wear dry-cleaned clothes? (Select one) (Zero points if green dry cleaning.)

0 days	1 day	2 days	3 days	4 days	5 days	6 days	7 days
0 pts	4 pts	6 pts	8 pts	10 pts	12 pts	14 pts	16 pts

Your "Rub" danger score

1–20	21–40	41–60	61+
Nice and comfy	Feeling itchy?	Too close for comfort	Rubbed the wrong way

Not-So-Natural Fabric

We've all heard the question, "What are you wearing?" Most likely you've never answered, "Petroleum, pesticides, perfluorochemicals, and antimony, with cadmium accessories." Yet in most cases, that would be the honest answer.

Modern clothing is far more complicated than simply considering the designer on the label or the sale price. Stop for a moment and read the tag on the shirt or pants you're wearing right now. For once, don't worry about the size. Instead look at the list of fibers that make up the garment. It's likely that you'll see a blend of fabrics—for example, 97 percent rayon and 3 percent spandex or 65 percent polyester and 35 percent cotton. If you take an inventory of your entire closet, you may find a few fabric names or blends you don't even recognize.

Most of us still tend to think of our clothing from the perspectives of fashion and fit:

- Does it look good?
- Do we look good wearing it?

But there are two other questions we should always ask in regards to our clothing and other fabrics:

- What is it made of?
- What is it doing to our body?

Ever since humans discovered that fibers could protect the body better than animal skins, fabric has been an important part of our lives. For thousands of years the four staple fabric fibers were flax, wool, cotton, and silk—all products created from natural sources. Natural fibers do have their limitations, though. Cotton and linens wrinkle, silk requires delicate handling, wool shrinks and can be scratchy. So people were understandably enthusiastic when advancements in technology over the last century allowed the clothing industry to trade in natural fabrics—and their limitations—for synthetic fabrics.

These new man-made materials, such as nylon and polyester, provided wrinkle and stain resistance, antimicrobial properties, and flame resistance. Today, however, we're discovering that the benefits of synthetic fibers are often outweighed by the health hazards they pose. The development of man-made material has necessitated the invention of thousands of new chemicals, only a few of which have undergone even the most basic human health screening. The chemicals, which now have direct contact with our bodies, can be absorbed through the skin, inhaled as they evaporate from the fabric, or—in the case of infants—sucked on and swallowed as they teethe.

In a way, our clothes have become as highly processed as our food; both have moved from healthy and natural to convenient and toxic.

Plastic Pants

To understand what potentially toxic chemicals exist in or on our clothes—and, therefore, in our bodies—we need to consider how synthetic clothes are made.

Today virtually all examples of synthetic fiber manufacturing are hazardous to our health. For example, the cancer-causing polyvinyl chloride (PVC) is widely agreed to be the most objectionable of all plastics, and yet we still see it being made softer and more flexible through the addition of toxic plasticizers—typically phthalates, which can wreak havoc on our hormones, as well—for use in clothing.

In another example, polyester is manufactured from petroleum products through a process that involves the use of a metal called antimony. Extended exposure to antimony can adversely affect the heart, digestive system, eyes, skin, and lungs.[1]

Perfluorochemicals, or PFCs, which include the nonstick additive Teflon®, are added to fabrics for durability, stain resistance, and wrinkle resistance. PFCs are extremely persistent in the body because they cannot be metabolized, or broken down. They accumulate in the cells and have been linked to reproductive and developmental toxicity as well as cancers of the liver and bladder. Clothing labeled as "no iron" will typically contain PFCs. Unfortunately, growing numbers of school children and workers are required to wear no-iron uniforms every day.

The increased use of petrochemical plastics and other synthetic fibers in such products as clothing and upholstery has increased the flammability of these products, making it necessary to impose

Simple Solution:
Cut down on the wrinkle-free materials. Five minutes of ironing will spare you from a lifetime of PFC exposure.

additional chemical treatments to meet fire standards. The most common class of chemicals used to protect against fire are halogenated flame retardants (HFRs), which have been linked to thyroid disruption, reproductive and neurodevelopmental problems, immune suppression, and—in some animal studies—cancer.[2]

In the past, most fabric dyes were derived from natural sources such as plants, animals, or minerals. That era ended a century and a half ago. Today, there is much heavier use of metals such as cadmium, cobalt, and antimony in the manufacture of dyes. Coloring is the most complex aspect in fabric production. *When* the dyes are added—whether before weaving, after the fabric is weaved into bolts, or as part of the final production—helps determine both the effects of the dyes on the environment and how they will be released over time from the completed garment, carpeting, or other products.

Shop Smart

By choosing fabrics made from natural fibers, you'll avoid at least some of the chemicals we just discussed. As an additional benefit, natural fabrics tend to "breathe" better than synthetic fibers and often wick moisture away from the body.

Whenever possible, stay away from the following fabrics:

- Acrylic
- Polyester
- Acetate
- Triacetate
- Nylon
- Anything labeled "static resistant," "wrinkle resistant," "permanent press," "no iron," "stain-proof," or "moth repellant"

Seek out these more natural alternatives:[3]

- Cotton
- Linen
- Wool
- Cashmere
- Silk
- Hemp

Keep in mind that not even natural fibers are completely safe or environmentally sustainable. According to one crop production report, the cotton industry is one of the top five users of herbicides in the United States.[4] Although organic cotton can be difficult to find in department stores, for infant clothing and your own wardrobe basics it may be worth your time to track down fabrics that are documented to have been grown and harvested without the use of pesticides.

Simple Solution:
Make certain your body is wrapped in safe, natural material for at least a third of the day by purchasing pajamas and bedding made from organic cotton.

The Smell of Clean?

Every day we see a television commercial featuring an ecstatic mother who is never harried or stressed. Why is she smiling with that happy glint in her eye? Her nose is buried in freshly washed laundry that smells like a "mountain spring."

If you've ever sat next to a real mountain spring, you know it doesn't smell like perfumed laundry.

Nevertheless, we're led to believe that this woman on the commercial is a better mom because her laundry looks cleaner and smells fresher than that of mothers using other leading brands.

Amazing.

What's *truly* amazing is that we're buying the potentially dangerous products she's peddling. Merchandisers bank on our love of scent. What most people don't think about is the origins of those scents. That whiff of "mountain spring" comes from scientists—dressed in protective white lab coats and masks—who wheel around on little stools, mixing compounds until they've found a way to reproduce "natural" smells through the use of chemicals.

> That whiff of "mountain spring" comes from scientists . . . mixing compounds until they've found a way to reproduce "natural" smells through the use of chemicals.

Although we may be tricked by artificial smells, our cells aren't. The skin is the body's largest organ, and contrary to popular opinion, it's not just a barrier that shields us against outside invaders. In fact, it's similar to a fine mesh that allows tiny particles to pass in and out of the body. Think of the nicotine patch that doses the wearer with chemicals that alter the body and mind. What's the difference between that and the residue that detergents and dryer sheets leave behind, coating your clothing and touching your skin? We may not be able to see it happening and we might prefer to ignore it, but those chemical residues are impacting our bodies.

But it's not just the fragrances that lurk in our clothes.

Something Stinks in the State of Fragrance

Until the twentieth century, fragrances and perfumes were made from natural substances like roots, barks, flowers, and berries, all of which were soaked in water and animal fats to produce fragrant oils.[5]

Today, however, the National Academy of Science reports that up to 95 percent of the chemicals used to make fragrances are synthetic compounds derived from petroleum, including known toxins capable of causing cancer, birth defects, central nervous system disorders, and allergic reactions. Many of these chemicals are derived from benzene, one of the most carcinogenic chemicals known to mankind.[6]

Of particular concern is the fact that many of the toxic compounds used to manufacture fragrances can actually penetrate the womb and harm an unborn

Ask the Scientist

"Dr. Wentz, what is our best defense against the toxic world in which we live?"

The best way to defend yourself against the toxins we're exposed to in today's world is to be educated and aware of the dangers so you can avoid them.

Another powerful strategy is to train and trust your nose. Of all our senses, smell makes the most direct connection between the outside world and your brain. Volatile organic compounds (VOCs) such as artificial fragrances can enter the body through the nose by inhalation, the mouth by ingestion, or the skin by absorption. Exposure to fragrances produces various combinations of sensory organ pathology, pulmonary damage, decreases in lung capacity, and increased symptoms of neurotoxicity.

Fragrances are among the most common causes of allergic reactions, including contact dermatitis. The Institute of Medicine has placed fragrance in the same category as secondhand smoke in triggering asthma in adults and school-aged children.[7]

Your nose can alert you immediately when you are exposed to toxic substances. For example, the moment you walk into a beauty parlor, your olfactory cells will warn you that toxic VOCs

child. Exposure to chemical fragrances found in many cosmetics may damage the reproductive system of a human male fetus as early as eight weeks into the pregnancy.[8]

Today fragrances are added to thousands of products, including health and beauty aids, laundry soaps and conditioners, household cleaners, paper products, oils and solvents, drugs, candles, plastics, and even foods.

Detergents and fabric softeners described as "fragrance free" or "unscented" on the label may still contain fragrance-inducing chemicals. Such labels only imply that the product has no perceptible odor. A product labeled "unscented" often contains a masking fragrance introduced during the manufacturing process that neutralizes odors. Manufacturers aren't required to list a fragrance on the label if it is added to a product to mask or cover up the odor of other ingredients.

are present and within threatening proximity of your brain cells.

Some of the chemicals found in scented products are potentially hazardous through secondary mechanisms as well. For instance, acetone—used in hundreds of products—is considered to pose only a moderate health hazard itself. However, it can work in a synergistic manner with other materials to increase the liver toxicity of chemicals such as carbon tetrachloride, chloroform, and trichloroethylene. Acetone also appears to inhibit the metabolism and elimination of ethyl alcohol, thereby increasing its toxicity.[9]

This makes it very difficult for consumers to know exactly what they are exposing themselves to when using a specific product. But you can lessen your risk by slowly eliminating the laundry products you know contain added chemical fragrances. You can also be more confident with reputable "green" brands that have built their entire businesses on offering customers safer, natural alternatives.

The fragrance industry tells consumers that their chemicals have not been proven toxic. However, it doesn't take a scientist to recognize that chemically produced scents are dangerous to living things. Even a California schoolgirl was able to develop a science fair project that demonstrated the toxic effects of certain perfumes and colognes. She sprayed cotton balls with

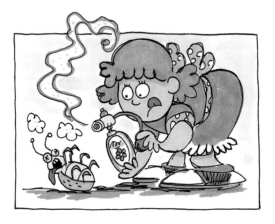

perfumes and colognes made by Calvin Klein, Polo, and others. Then she put the cotton balls into some cups, each with a live cricket, and sealed the cups with plastic food wrap secured with a rubber band. By timing how long it took the crickets to die, she determined that Calvin Klein was the most toxic perfume—death in eighty-four seconds.

The most toxic cologne was the appropriately named Axe brand.[10]

Ask yourself: If perfume or cologne can kill crickets in a matter of seconds, what damage can they do to someone who wears them all day long? Give extra thought to saturating your clothing and bedding—and more importantly, the clothing of your children—in similar chemical perfumes that are part of the "cleaning process."

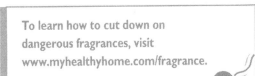

To learn how to cut down on dangerous fragrances, visit www.myhealthyhome.com/fragrance.

Your laundry is one everyday part of your life in which you can easily eliminate unnecessary chemicals. Nontoxic, natural detergents are readily available in many supermarkets and most natural food stores. Reusable cloth dryer sheets or non-PVC dryer balls—which help reduce static cling—can be found online. At the very, very least, you can select unscented or lightly scented mainstream laundry products.

Simple Solution:
Use one-half cup of white vinegar in place of fabric softener in the washer to reduce static cling and soften clothing. *Important note: Never combine vinegar and bleach in the same load; toxic fumes can result.*

Our cotton sheets should not smell like lavender, and our jeans should not smell like mountain air unless we live in the mountains. We need to retrain our noses to appreciate the true scent of clean—which is no scent at all. When you smell smoke in your home, you know there is danger. So when you smell those fragrant sheets or that cloying cologne, you should know to run like your life depends on it.

Because it does.

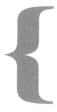

> We need to retrain our noses to appreciate the true scent of clean—which is no scent at all.

The Mysteries of Dry Cleaning

What in the heck is dry cleaning?

The secret of how our clothes get processed at the dry cleaners is something few of us care to unravel. After all, the point is for our clothes to *look* clean and crisp and that we don't have to do the work required to get them that way. We've come to rely on having professionally laundered clothing hanging in our closet, neatly pressed and ready to grab off the hanger. Besides, it's relatively cheap for such a convenient service.

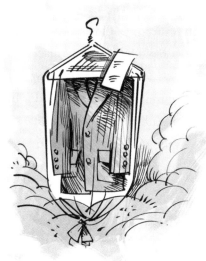

The problem is that most of us don't have a clue about what's involved in the process of dry cleaning.

The first irony here is that the process isn't dry. The second is that the process doesn't leave your clothes clean—it leaves them polluted with chemicals. "Dry cleaning" is actually a wet process wherein stain-removing agents are added to a machine that looks like a washing machine. It is called "dry" cleaning because the cleaning agents aren't water soluble.

Perchloroethylene (perc), a solvent and volatile organic compound (VOC), is the strong-smelling cleaning agent that's most commonly used, and it dries quickly. It has the *appearance* of water but has a consistency similar to gasoline. Perc soaks into your clothing, which then goes through a washing process to remove what we think of as soil.

But here's the kicker: The cleaning process that removes the dirt does *not* remove the dry cleaning solution. Your garments are still soiled—not with mustard, coffee, or sweat—but with toxic chemicals.

If, as you read this, you are wearing clothes that have been dry cleaned, you are being exposed to perchloroethylene because it has been absorbed by the fabric and does not wash out. The health effects of perc, especially when used over prolonged periods of time, are frightening. Long-term exposure can cause kidney and liver damage and has been proven in laboratories to cause cancer in animals.[11] Even short-term exposure has its risks, including dizziness, a rapid heart rate, headaches, and skin irritation.

A central nervous system depressant, perc can enter the body through the lungs and skin. In fact, exposure to perc can be measured via a breathalyzer test, much like alcohol. Stored in the fat, perc is released slowly into the bloodstream and can be detected for weeks after heavy exposure. One study on residential air quality in New Jersey examined the effect of bringing

{ When a chemical is proven dangerous, our government considers economic concerns first and public health hazards second. }

dry-cleaned clothes into the home. The study found that elevated levels of perc persisted for up to forty-eight hours. During that time, inhalation levels of perc increased two to six times for people in the exposed settings.[12]

Because of this danger, California and a few other U.S. states have ordered that perc be phased out by the year 2023. Considering that so many other states haven't taken *any* action to ban perc, California and states like it should be applauded. Yet their citizens are still looking at another decade or so of poisoning. It's hard to believe that even when a chemical is proven dangerous, our government considers economic concerns first and public health hazards second.

Give It Air

Does this mean you should resign yourself to looking wrinkled, stained, and frumpy?

No, the "slovenly professor" look isn't necessary. There are several things you can do to limit your exposure to perc or completely eliminate it from your life once and for all while still keeping your clothes and linens looking fresh.

First, you can reduce your risk by thoroughly airing out any dry-cleaned clothing or other household fabrics. You can do this by hanging it outside or placing it in the garage or a well-ventilated room with a way to sweep the chemicals *outside*.

Then give it the sniff test—if it still smells like the cleaners, air it out for another day or two.

You also can wear an undershirt or tank top underneath jackets or sweaters to reduce skin contact with perc-treated clothing. This yields the bonus of allowing

Simple Solution:
Unwrap and air out your dry-cleaned garments for at least two days in an exterior area, like a garage—never in a closet or bedroom.

you to wear the clothing additional times between cleaning. Thus, if your suit isn't dirty or smelly, don't send it to the cleaners. Just air it out and iron it, because the cleaning agent is still there.

Use Greener Cleaners

Several environmentally responsible and less toxic alternatives to perc have recently emerged, including paraffin-based agents, propylene glycol ethers, and liquid CO_2 (carbon dioxide). And with states like California imposing increasingly stringent use restrictions on VOCs, it's likely that more and more dry cleaners will begin to offer these sensible substitutes.

Start by calling around or looking online (using keywords like "eco-friendly dry cleaners") for cleaners in your area who employ paraffin-based cleaning agents, such as DF 2000®, Pure Dry®, and EcoSolv®, or who use any of the propylene glycol ethers marketed as Rynex®, Impress®, Gen-X®, and Solvair®. You can also look for cleaners who have introduced a new "wet-cleaning" technology. This process uses water along with biodegradable detergents to produce a solvent in a computer-controlled process that preserves fabric integrity through humidity-controlled drying.

And if you're fortunate enough to have a cleaner in your area who uses liquid CO_2, look no further. Liquid CO_2 is effective, nontoxic, and easy on the environment, making it an excellent dry-cleaning choice.

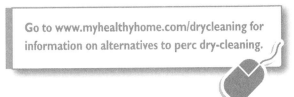

Go to www.myhealthyhome.com/drycleaning for information on alternatives to perc dry-cleaning.

Do It Yourself

Labels sometimes lie.

For instance, my size 34 jeans are really size 35, but the company labeled them smaller so I would feel good about myself. And it works. I don't buy "truthful" brands with which I can't fit into a size 34.

Labels also lie when it comes to instructions for care and cleaning. Clothing labeled "dry clean only" can often be laundered at home after it has been dry cleaned just one time. What's more, many natural fabrics—even wool and silk—can be gently laundered at home without them ever having been dry cleaned. You can launder these kinds of fabrics with a gentle detergent on a delicate wash cycle with cold water and then line dry or use a low setting in a tumble dryer. For seriously delicate fabrics like silk or cashmere, hand wash them in cold water with mild soap and then air dry.

There's always some risk of damage, shrinkage, or color loss, but are you more concerned about damaging your clothes or your long-term health? Dry cleaning may be one everyday behavior for which we can do more than reduce our exposure to toxins. We may be able to rid ourselves of it entirely.

Constrictive Clothing

If you're like most people, you put a lot more thought into how you dress in the morning than you do about getting undressed at night. But have you stopped to look at your body after slipping off those socks, wriggling out of those pants, or unsnapping that bra at the end of the day?

Those angry red lines on your skin after you've removed a snug piece of clothing should be viewed as a serious red flag.

Constrictive fabric acts as a tourniquet, hindering critical lymphatic circulation. Lymphatic flow is a delicate process that carries nutrients, removes waste, and fights germs throughout the body. Yet as important as the lymphatic system is to your health, it does not have a powerful pump—like your heart—to keep it flowing.

{ Those angry red lines on your skin after you've removed a snug piece of clothing should be viewed as a serious red flag. }

Instead, slight muscle contractions and even your breathing help circulate lymphatic fluid. My first lymphatic massage, received a few years ago at Sanoviv Medical Institute, was a wake-up call. The massage involved only the lightest touch to help stimulate my lymphatic system's detoxification function. I remember being surprised by just how gentle the massage was, and I came to the realization that if the lymphatic process really is this subtle, then constrictive clothing can easily keep our lymphatic system from doing its critical job.

So Loosen the Lingerie

TRUE OR FALSE? Women who come from cultures in which bra wearing is the norm are more likely to get breast cancer than women who don't.

The answer: True.

Many factors come into play, including diet, levels of stress, body weight, lifestyle, and childbearing practices, but the fact is that women of other cultures are more than just "liberated." The lymph flow pumps up along the rib cage and across the breast area. Wearing a snug, ill-fitting bra is like wearing a blood pressure cuff that's been pumped up tight and may be cutting off a delicately maintained circulation that is vital to the immune system.

This isn't a call for a mass bra burning, but be honest with yourself about whether or not you're wearing something too tight. Many bra-fitting experts advise women to move to a smaller bra circumference for better lift and support. Before you plunk down half a paycheck on the latest lacy contraption, check to see if the bra leaves red marks on your skin or if you can't comfortably fit a finger or two between your bra band and your back.

If it feels too tight, it is—no matter what your fitting expert says. Go up a size or two and feel good about what you're doing for your lymphatic system and long-term health.

Simple Solution:
Reduce stress on your lymphatic system for at least a few extra hours a day by removing your bra when you're in the privacy of your home.

Men, our bodies need adequate circulation, too. And we can be slaves to our egos when it comes to clothing.

How many of us have been known to refuse to budge on our pant size, despite having gained a few pounds? We also have watches, belts, shirt collars, and ties to contend with. Go down another layer. Are your socks tight enough to leave impressions after you take them off? What about your underwear?

Many of us put on a pound or two every year, and too often we try to continue wearing clothes that are the same size as what we wore in high school. A report from Cornell University found that 67 percent of men were buying and wearing shirts with a neck size smaller than the actual circumference of their necks. Those same men then tied their ties too tight, attempting to match the collar size of the shirt.[13]

It's not just our lymphatic systems that we're choking. Dr. Susan Watkins, leader of the Cornell study, suggests that tightness around the neck constricts the arteries and decreases the flow of oxygenated blood to the brain and the sensory organs of the head—the nose, ears, and eyes. Subjects in the study were asked to tell researchers when a light, flickering at increased speeds, appeared to become constant. The men with tight collars reported the poorest visual discrimination.

The pressure on the jugular veins in the neck can also lead to increased fluid pressure inside the eye. Though loosening the tie and collar allows the pressure within the eye to return to normal within minutes, tight neckwear can certainly introduce a risk of increased intraocular pressure, which is the most important risk factor leading to glaucoma and other eye disorders.[14]

Farther down the body, the biggest problem comes from pants that are too small. One doctor who looked at approximately two hundred male patients with unexplained stomach problems—such as heartburn, bloating, and belching—found that the symptoms were directly related to poorly fitting pants. His measurements showed a discrepancy of at least three inches between the men's actual waistlines and the waistbands of their pants.[15]

{ A report from Cornell University found that 67 percent of men were buying and wearing shirts with a neck size smaller than the actual circumference of their necks. }

Many men don't even *realize* they've outgrown their old size, unconsciously shifting the pants lower on their hips to avoid their expanding bellies. For many others, it's a matter of ego. The men just don't want to admit to themselves or their significant others that they're too large around the waist to fit into the pant sizes they've always worn.

The answer is easy: Men should either try on and buy their own pants or fess up to the women who shop for them. Remember, nobody can see the tags on our clothing. What they *can* see is that our pants are bursting at the seams. Men who are wearing the correct size are more comfortable and look better for it.

Simple Solution:
Purchase your clothing based on how it fits, not what size is on the label.

Another cause of constriction among weekend warriors is the increased use of neoprene "warm pants" made to prevent muscular injury. Designed to stimulate blood circulation by massage and to counteract swelling by compression, these "tourniquets" can cause deep vein blood clots, and such damage could be much more serious than the pulled muscles they're meant to prevent.[16]

The bottom line is that being realistic about your clothing size is important for both your short-term comfort and your long-term wellness.

> Jumping on a mini-trampoline—a rebounder—is another great way to pump your lymphatic system. Get more information at www.myhealthyhome.com/rebounder.

What's in a Mattress?

Like Goldilocks in her fabled visit to the three bears' house, we all search for a bed that's "just right" for providing a good night's sleep.

But comfort isn't the only thing to consider when it comes to a mattress. Whether you're in the market for a new mattress set or contending with an inherited relic, you should know what you're getting when you get into bed.

The average furniture store will have two basic types of mattresses in stock:

- Memory foam
- Innerspring

The key material of concern for both types of mattresses is polyurethane foam, a product so flammable that the insurance industry calls it "solid gasoline." Fire-retardant chemicals are applied to most mattresses to combat polyurethane's tendency to explode at the slightest spark.

Until 2005 the synthetic foam used in mattresses was typically saturated in highly toxic fire-retardant chemicals called polybrominated diphenyl ethers (PBDEs). These global pollutants, still in use in many home electronics, build up in the blood and tissues of people and wildlife, affecting their brains and reproductive systems.[17] Although the use of this dangerous chemical in mattresses has since been phased out in the United States, many people are still exposed to it through their old mattresses. Meanwhile, federal flammability standards have grown even tougher, which means mattress manufacturers have been forced to find new fire retardants to keep the flames at bay.

So nearly any mattress you buy in the United States will have at least some flame-retardant properties. The systems used to combat flammability vary from company to company, none of which are required to tell us what chemicals have been used in their mattresses. Many manufacturers are likely using antimony, a dangerous heavy metal we learned about earlier, and other brominated fire retardants that are known to disrupt hormone activity and interfere with brain function. Surveys have shown that these chemicals are steadily accumulating in the bodies of our children and grandchildren. Flame retardants have also been developed from things like salt, clay, and Kevlar.

Fortunately, you do have a few options for catching healthier ZZZs. If you're looking to buy a new mattress any time soon, organic mattresses made with natural latex and/or naturally flame-resistant wool are a good option. That said, finding a truly organic mattress can be difficult. There are many mattress companies that claim to make natural mattresses, but they are likely treated with some pretty nasty chemical flame retardants. If you're going to make the considerable investment to purchase an organic mattress, you need to be prepared to ask a lot of questions.

Simple Solution:
Whenever you launder your sheets, open your windows and leave your mattress exposed in order to allow your bed to off-gas for the day.

If you must purchase a new synthetic mattress, consider unwrapping it and allowing it to off-gas outside for at least a few days before using it. You could also add a natural latex mattress topper to provide a healthier barrier between your body and any toxic materials. Remember, you'll likely spend up to a third of your life lying on your mattress, so do whatever you can to have a restful night without risking your long-term health.

Go to www.myhealthyhome.com/mattress to get more information about safer bed options.

Chapter 2
The Body Electric!

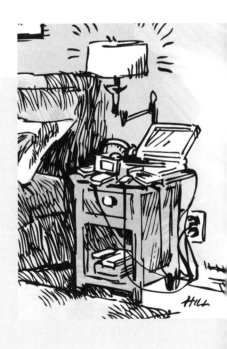

We cannot see it, taste it, or feel it, but every day we are barraged by electromagnetic radiation produced by many of the conveniences of the modern world. From the alarm clock on the nightstand to the Wi-Fi router in the office, we are continuously adding invisible energy fields throughout our home, and with them, we are increasing the risk of serious health consequences.

We've become the guinea pigs in a massive technology industry experiment.

QUIZ How Toxic Is Your Home?   Scores

1. How many gadgets are plugged in within four feet of the head of your bed? Be sure to consider alarm clocks, mp3 docking stations, mobile phone chargers, baby monitors, lamps, etc. (3 pts each)

2. While you sleep, where is your mobile phone? (Select one)
   ☐ Under your pillow (8 pts)   ☐ In the room but not reachable (4 pts)
   ☐ Right next to the bed (6 pts) ☐ In another room (0 pts)

3. How many major electrical appliances are near your bed? Consider fuse boxes, electric heating units, electric water heaters, air conditioning units, televisions, etc. Don't forget what's on the other side of the wall. (6 pts each)

4. Do you use an electric blanket?

Never	Sometimes in the winter	Always in the winter	Always
0 pts	3 pts	7 pts	12 pts

Your "Electric" danger score

1–8	9–16	17–24	25+
Energy-efficient	Slightly charged	High voltage	Zapped

The Ying and Yang of EMFs

Like most of you, I don't actually remember learning about electromagnetic fields (EMFs) back when I was fourteen, but assuming that I did, I'm pretty sure I didn't appreciate their beauty and potential danger like I do now.

All matter is made of atoms, which are composed of negatively charged electrons flying around a positively charged nucleus of protons and neutrons. Think of the sun as the nucleus and the planets as the electrons held in orbit by attraction. These charged particles produce electric and magnetic fields. On the largest scale, the universe itself simply would not exist if it weren't for these forces and fields. The electromagnetism of life is not only all around us, it's all *through* us.

Everything that exists does so due to the balance between the charged particles—negative and positive, attraction and repulsion. Every drop of water in the ocean, every grain of sand in the desert, every blade of grass on the prairie—all of it is involved in a delicate dance of opposites.[1]

With the rise of human technology, a wide range of new EMFs has been introduced to the planet's surface. Every electronic gadget, power line, household appliance, computer, and power outlet is creating an EMF of its very own. Many of these man-made EMFs are of a higher magnitude than is found in nature and are different enough to have novel effects on our biological systems.

Our world is swamped with manmade EMFs, and the earth's life forms—as well as the air, water, and soil—may be suffering both positive and negative effects, no pun intended. Denying the power of EMFs is like denying the power of gravity—they're both invisible forces that have very real, if sometimes subtle, effects on life itself. Although we're only beginning to understand what high-tech EMF pollution may be doing to alter our health, let's take a closer look at several ranges of EMFs we find in our homes, identify the potential risks, and learn how we can minimize them.

If you are a typical member of modern society, you have a seriously wired nightstand. Alarm clocks, lamps, baby monitors, cell phone chargers—all of the things we mentioned in the chapter quiz—sit next to your bed, plugged in just a few feet from your brain during the hours you lie asleep. And every gadget is creating its own electromagnetic field with which your body—and all of its individual cells—must contend.

The EMFs we're talking about are similar to those found under major power lines that were linked to cancer clusters and dominated the news in the 1970s until we got tired of hearing about it.[2] News is only interesting when it's new. Yet you don't have to live under a high-voltage power line to be subjected every minute of the day to man-made EMF radiations that may have negative effects on your moods and metabolism.

But why is that a problem?

The human body is powered and regulated by extremely complex chemical and electromagnetic systems of its own. Electromagnetic fields can seriously disrupt the normal electromagnetic energies of the body.

EMFs created by household gadgets—such as alarm clocks, lights, and electric heaters—are examples of extremely low frequency (ELF) fields, with frequencies from 3 to 300 cycles per second, or 300 Hertz (Hz). Other technologies, such as computer monitors, security alarms, and antitheft devices, create intermediate frequency fields ranging from 300 Hz to 10 million Hz (or 10 MHz). Depending on how strong and how close they are, these fields can induce currents in the human body that produce a range of biological effects.[3]

EMFs can be found throughout your home, including wiring and outlets, as well as anything that's plugged into those outlets—whether they're turned on or not. The early consensus was that ELF fields associated with normal household living do not constitute a short-term or a long-term health hazard.[4] However, most of these opinions are based on outdated exposure limits designed to minimize the chance of thermal effects—in other words, that the radiation would actually heat (or burn) your body's tissues.

However, early research did not look at whether limits are conservative enough to protect against possible *nonthermal* effects, which are the less obvious but potentially significant changes to your cellular function that could cause long-term damage. It's like saying that if people weren't immediately killed by a nuclear blast, they wouldn't need to worry about the long-term effects of the fallout.

Several recent studies support the existence of adverse non-thermal effects from ELF fields,[5] and others have revealed an association with childhood cancer.[6] Cancer was first associated with exposure to electromagnetic fields in 1979, when investigators reported that specific children dying from cancer resided in homes that researchers believed had been exposed to higher ELF fields than those of healthy children.[7] Other research has implicated ELF field exposure with a host of adverse effects, ranging from adult melanoma[8] to neurodegenerative disease[9] to miscarriage.[10]

It all comes down to a simple question: Why expose yourself to a potential risk if you don't have to?

Although you can't rip the wiring out of your house, you *can* make

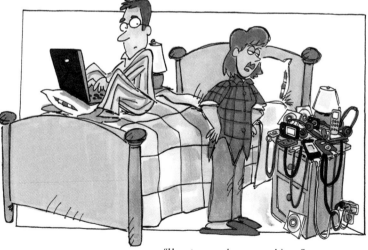

"Houston, we have a problem."

some easy changes to your habits to reduce your ELF and IF field exposure. First, you can do your best to remove electronics from the one room where you spend up to a third of your time—the bedroom. This means clearing your nightstand of any unnecessary gadgets, so charge your iPod and cell phone elsewhere. Distancing your headboard from lamps is also a good idea, though this may be inconvenient for many people. If you can't live without your electric blanket in the winter, warm it up before bedtime, then unplug it prior to climbing into bed. Finally, move your bed entirely if it is situated above or beside a

Simple Solution:

Unplug your electronic gadgets and appliances when they aren't being used.

high ELF field generator like a fuse box or an electric heating or cooling unit.

One gadget you may want to introduce to your home is a Gauss meter, which detects and measures EMFs. This relatively inexpensive device will help

Visit www.myhealthyhome.com/meter for more information on Gauss meters and how to use them.

Cellular Truths

EMFs and Cells

The forces of attraction and repulsion between elementary particles—as well as the fields they use to communicate with each other—can provide us with clues about the effects EMFs have on cells.

The truth is that today's conventional medicine has no accepted biological model for the mechanism by which low-level electromagnetic radiation can cause damage to the human body. Yet there are some strong candidates.[11]

1. We know that calcium ions, and possibly magnesium ions, can be removed from cell membranes by electromagnetic fields. This would make the membranes more porous to other materials and more likely to tear and leak.

2. DNA fragmentation, which is seen in cells exposed to EMFs at frequencies used by mobile phones, may be caused by leakage of important enzymes from the lysosomes inside the cell. When this happens in reproductive cells there would be a reduction in fertility and increased genetic disorders in future generations.

you identify the biggest EMF problem areas in your home so you can avoid, lessen, or eliminate them.

A Higher Power

With technology advancing at breakneck speed, society now must contend with an even stronger source of EMF exposure— cellular phones and Wi-Fi (wireless networks). These technologies, along with microwave ovens, radios, and televisions, are generators of radio frequencies from 30 MHz to 300 billion Hz (or 300 GHz).

Microwave technology, which is part of the radiofrequency (RF) spectrum, was first developed by the German military during World War II. Soldiers who had gathered around radar units to warm themselves were later found to develop illnesses, including cancer. Nowadays, with the soaring popularity of wireless technologies such as cell phones and Wi-Fi networks, our exposure to microwave fields is nearly constant.

If it sounds a little scary, that's because it is.

Almost twenty years after cellular communication was introduced to the global market, we are reaching the end of the latency period for cancers to appear, and the scientific evidence is mounting that cell phone use *is* associated with the development of serious adverse health effects. We'll be revisiting the impact that modern technology has on our health in more detail in chapter 11, "High-Tech, High-Risk." We'll also take a closer look in chapter 8 at the dangers of exposure to microwave ovens.

3. Calcium is perhaps the most important signaling molecule in the cell. If calcium ions leak into the cytosol, they will act as a metabolic stimulant. The expected results would be an acceleration in cell proliferation and growth of cancerous tumors.

All living cells employ electromagnetism for the most basic functions of metabolism and growth. However, major changes in the strength of fields and shifts of radiation frequencies—which we are seeing in our technological age—may be severely disrupting cell function, especially in metabolically active tissue and developing organs in children.

The question is not whether EMFs affect cells. Rather, it is how *much* they do and how hazardous those effects are to the health of the cells and the body.

Chapter 3
Sleepytime

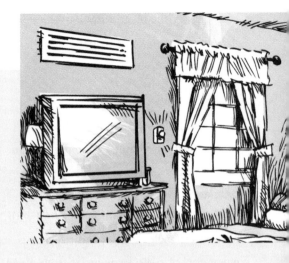

Adequate sleep is critical for maintaining good health, but it's often the first thing we allow to slide when life gets in the way. The dog knows her bedtime—though the neighbor's dog doesn't seem to—yet we humans act as if we've outsmarted our need for sleep.

Most of us make a half-hearted attempt at showing up at our beds only after we're too exhausted to do anything else. But lying down doesn't automatically yield rejuvenating sleep. While getting to the bedroom on time can be a challenge, once we do get there several key factors will determine whether or not we are able to get both the *quality* and *quantity* of sleep we need. And just like legitimate work involves more than punching a time clock, legitimate rest involves our whole being—not just the body.

QUIZ

How Toxic Is Your Home?   Scores

1. How well do you typically sleep? (Select one)

☐ Rarely wake (0 pts)   ☐ Toss and turn (8 pts)
☐ Wake up once or twice a night (2 pt)   ☐ I'm awake more than
☐ Wake up several times a night (4 pts)   I'm asleep (10 pts)

2. How light is your room during the hours you sleep?

Pitch black   Bright enough to read

| 0 pts | 2 pts | 4 pts | 6 pts | 8 pts | 10 pts |

3. Do you need a blaring alarm clock to wake up on weekdays? Yes_____ (5 pts)

4. Do you need a stimulant like caffeine in the morning to function? Yes_____(6 pts)

Your "Sleep" danger score

1–7	8–14	15–21	22+
Sleeping soundly	Rested but not revived	Nearing a rude awakening	A complete nightmare

I'll Sleep When I'm Dead

I confess, I'm a guilty party when it comes to rest.

I have a demanding career, want to spend time with my family and friends, and have sports and hobbies I love, including indoor soccer games that are sometimes scheduled at 11 p.m. I simply don't want to miss out on the fun! My philosophy is to never miss an opportunity to experience something new.

So I'm usually worried that I might be missing something fantastic when I'm asleep. Whether trying to complete an important report at work or fitting in late-night socializing with friends, it's easy to give up an hour or two of rest in order to get more of everything done.

But even if shortchanging our ZZZs doesn't kill us right away, without optimal sleep, we cannot be at our best, physically or mentally. Nature gives our bodies a built-in signal that tells us to begin slowing in preparation for complete rest. Think of it as our forced "time out," without which we'd become exhausted or ill.

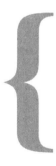

{ In the typical adult, even a week of getting two to three hours less than the optimum amount of sleep needed each night seriously undermines mood, alertness, and performance. }

Sleep holds the reins of our body's temperature, blood pressure, secretion of hormones, brain activity, and many more functions. The body needs sleep or meditative periods in order to process information, make sense of what we've been bombarded with during the day, and store it away in memory. In the typical adult, even a week of getting two to three hours less than the optimum amount of sleep needed each night seriously undermines mood, alertness, and performance.

If the brain isn't allowed time to reboot, we'll quickly experience serious memory problems. And longer-term sleep loss is pure torture to the body. It may hasten the onset of diabetes, high blood pressure, and memory loss, or it could worsen these conditions if they already exist.

Sleep's most important function may be the time it gives your body for cellular repair. That's why it's so important to take twice-daily multivitamin and mineral supplements, with an emphasis on minerals in the supplement you take with your evening meal. Even the *Journal of the American Medical Association* finally published a study that states that everyone should be taking a daily vitamin and mineral supplement.[1]

To increase effectiveness, take a product that separates the vitamins and minerals and provides much higher doses than outdated recommended daily allowances. A high quality vitamin product will provide important antioxidants, so take the majority in the morning to provide more protection during the day when your body is exposed to the greatest demands and stresses. Minerals are critically needed during cell building and repair, so you may want to take more of those in the evening to make them readily available during sleep. Coincidentally, some minerals—such as magnesium—also have a calming effect.

Simple Solution:
Take a mineral supplement with your evening meal to aid in cellular repair during sleep.

Your Bedroom Forecast

Periods of sleep—alternating with periods of activity—are important because every one of the almost 100 trillion cells in your body has its own "inner clock" with cycles that correspond to the passing of the twenty-four-hour cycle. Just how well that inner clock works, though, can depend on the quality of your sleeping environment. For a truly restful and restorative night's sleep, we cannot ignore the lighting and temperature in the bedroom.

Don't Let There Be Light

During most of mankind's existence, humans have been creatures of the daytime, rarely active at night due to the inherent dangers that lurk in the darkness. Today, with our access to inexpensive lighting sources, we are 24/7 creatures—working, playing, traveling, and eating at all hours of the day and night. But our bodies still naturally prepare for the semi- or unconscious state we call "sleep."

And we still need darkness to sleep well.

For awareness of light, we have light-sensitive ganglion cells in the retinas of our eyes that have nothing to do with seeing. When the light of day fades, they send a message to our brains that it's time to prepare for sleep, which means it's time for the pineal gland to begin producing the hormone *melatonin*. Melatonin is called the "hormone of darkness" because it regulates the sleep-wake cycle in humans, causing drowsiness, lowering body temperature, slowing metabolic functions, and otherwise putting the body into sleep mode.

Helping to regulate sleep and waking cycles may be a major function of melatonin, but it serves other purposes as well. It is a powerful antioxidant that can cross the blood-brain barrier and other cell membranes to help protect against free radicals. These unstable organic molecules can damage our cells and create oxidative stress, chain reactions that are linked to aging and degenerative disease. Melatonin also influences the immune system and helps to protect against infectious disease.

Simple Solution:

Take a melatonin supplement before bed to help promote your body's natural sleep process.

It appears that melatonin production can even affect a woman's risk of breast cancer. Researchers found that women who were totally blind had a 36 percent lower risk of breast cancer than sighted women.[2] Due to their lack of light perception, blind women typically produce higher levels of melatonin than their sighted counterparts. Lower melatonin production may also be the

> Just a flash of light in the middle of the night is enough to signal the pineal gland that the night is ending and it's time to get up...melatonin production is immediately ramped down.

reason women who work night shifts were found to have significantly higher incidence rates of cancer and other disorders.[3]

Just a flash of light in the middle of the night is enough to signal the pineal gland that the night is ending and it's time to get up—whether it is or not. Melatonin production is immediately ramped down. So if you have to make a trip to the bathroom, avoid turning on the light, if possible.

Recent studies indicate that melatonin is most sensitive to light in the blue range, which, unfortunately, is the color of light used in many electronic gadgets from alarm clocks and clock radios to cell phones, DVD players, cable modems, and game consoles. If you want a good, restful period of sleep, all of those appliances should be banished from the bedroom, or at least turned away from the bed.

Simple Solution:
Buy nightlights, alarm clocks, and other bedroom electronics that are illuminated with red light, which is less disturbing to melatonin production than white or blue light.

Don't forget about the light that comes from outside your bedroom. Streetlamps, car headlights, your neighbor's porch light, and even moonlight can all encroach on your sleep as they stream through your bedroom windows. Because of this, window treatments serve a more valuable purpose than mere interior decoration. Whether you install blinds or drapes, ensure that your bedroom windows are fully covered to block out all light pollution.

What is the best temperature for sleeping?

Rather than identifying a specific range, experts agree that whatever temperature the sleeper finds comfortable will have a positive effect on how well and how long he or she will snooze. When your body becomes uncomfortably hot or cold, the brain signals a wake-up call.

But for most people, cooler is better.

Why?

According to H. Craig Heller, Ph.D., professor of biology at Stanford University, your body's set point for temperature naturally declines during sleep. "Think of it as the internal thermostat," he said. In fact, a slight drop in body temperature helps induce sleep. If it's too hot, the body must work to achieve this set point; and when the body is working, it is not resting.[4]

Ralph Downey III, Ph.D., chief of sleep medicine at Loma Linda University, also found that the comfort level of your bedroom temperature affects the quality of rapid eye movement (REM) sleep, the stage in which you dream.[5]

> **Simple Solution:**
> Take a warm bath before bed. Your body's natural drop in temperature afterward will help you fall asleep.

Dr. Wentz recommends sleeping in a room cool enough that you will want to cover most of your body with at least a sheet, which also blocks neurotransmitters in your skin from being stimulated by light.

In Search of Clean Air

The old tradition of saying "God bless you" or "Gesundheit" when another person sneezes is derived in part from an old folk tale that claims your spirit temporarily leaves the body during the involuntary outburst. The real danger, however, may not be the sneeze or exhale. In certain rooms of the house, we should be saying a prayer each time we *inhale*!

- Do you often feel sluggish in the morning, unable to focus through a foggy brain?
- Do you suffer from headaches, asthma, allergies, or congestion?

The air may be a culprit. Many rooms in modern homes have air that's stale, stagnant, and filled with chemical pollutants. This is especially a concern in the bedroom, where you're sucking down bad air by the lungful all night long.

You may remember or have read about the heavy layers of orange-grey haze that blanketed cities such as Los Angeles prior to 1970. Thanks to the Clean Air Act, we hear less about that kind of industrial air pollution today. Yet we still tend to think about pollution only when it's outside and far enough away that we can see it. We worry about breathing exhaust when we see great clouds of smoke pluming out of chimneys or while we sit in traffic jams. But the main source of air pollution is much closer to home.

It's actually *in* our homes.

{ We still tend to think about pollution only when it's outside and far enough away that we can see it . . . but the main source of air pollution is much closer to home. }

According to the Environmental Protection Agency (EPA), Americans spend 90 percent of their time indoors—at home or in offices.[6] And while we're there, we're breathing air that is usually two to five times more polluted with organic pollutants than outdoor air.[7] We don't need to ask how they got in, either. We paint, spritz, and spray these pollutants, also known as volatile organic compounds (VOCs), all over our homes.

Now we need to make them go away.

Physicians are beginning to recognize that our sensitivity to VOCs results in symptoms that mimic a cold or hay fever. Congestion, throat and eye irritation, headache, dizziness, and fatigue plague the most vulnerable family members—our children and the elderly. Some suffer from symptoms as severe as asthma attacks and other respiratory illnesses, and we try to deal with them through medication.

Rather than adding several lifelong prescription drugs to your family budget, why not try eliminating the possible causes?

Creating Fresh Air

Despite the severity of our indoor air situation, we really have only three remedies for improving air quality:

1. Get rid of the sources of pollution.
2. Dilute the pollution with cleaner air from an open window.
3. Clean the existing polluted air through filtering.

The "stuff" that we're trying to clean out of the air is typically made up of particulate matter and gaseous pollutants. Particulates include dust, smoke, pollen, and particles generated from combustion appliances as well as biological particles associated with tiny organisms such as dust mites, bacteria, and molds. Gaseous pollutants can come from combustion processes, but they also come from the use of products such as adhesives, paints, cleaning products, and pesticides.

Do you remember the perfumes and dry cleaning chemicals we talked about earlier?

The best way to reduce the risk of indoor air pollution is *not* through filtering or purifying but rather by controlling or eliminating the sources of the pollutants—products that are polluting the air unnecessarily. As much as you can, ditch the adhesives, cleaning products, and other such items. By minimizing them, you'll remarkably improve your home environment.

Making certain your home has adequate ventilation involving fresh outside air is the next most effective method of preventing noxious gases and particulates from accumulating. So often we're worried about the outside environment, checking for updates on whether our city is having a red day or a green day on the air quality scale. In reality, our indoor air *comes from* outdoor air, and once it's inside, it becomes even more polluted and much more concentrated.

For this reason, the air outside our home is consistently cleaner than the air inside.

One of your main concerns with a bedroom that has direct access to the bathroom is that there is also direct airflow between the two. Without substantial airflow through open windows or efficient exhaust vents, the products used in the bathroom—such as perfumes, nail polishes and removers, and hairsprays—accumulate in an invisible cloud that floats in over the bed and hangs there.

You breathe these gases while you're sleeping.

So make sure you have an exhaust fan in your bathroom, and use it as much as possible. This will keep negative pressure in the bathroom so that the toxic products you use in there will be pulled outside instead of drifting into your sleeping area.

A last option for cleaning pollutants from your air is an air purifier. Numerous styles and quality levels are available on the market, each meant to control and remove allergens that trigger allergy, asthma, and other respiratory and immune system problems.

These devices are designed to remove certain types of pollutants, but *none* of them can effectively remove all particles and gases.

High-efficiency particulate arresting (HEPA) filter systems employ a great technology, but to work effectively, they often require a larger fan or motor capacity than is typically available in many residential home ventilation systems. If you opt for a HEPA filter purifier for your bedroom, be sure to consider motor noise, the air exchange rate, and the lifetime cost of replacing filters. A quality HEPA filter should be able to clean and exchange the air up to fifteen times per hour in an average-sized bedroom.

Keep in mind that standard HEPA filters capture particulates, not gases. So look for a HEPA air purifier that also features an activated carbon filter, which will remove some of the gaseous pollutants in the air as well.

To learn more about air purifiers, go to www.myhealthyhome.com/air.

Your Real Sleep Number

You've heard it since you were a child: You need eight hours of sleep to be at your best in the morning.

We all seem to strive for that magical number, and most of us fall short. When it comes to the amount of sleep we actually need, though, everyone is unique. Many of us require nine hours of rest to feel great, while others may perform well after just six and a half hours.

A simple weekend experiment will help tell you just how much sleep your body needs. Pay attention to how many hours you sleep after you go to bed on Friday night. Be sure it's *au naturale*—no sleep aids, caffeine, stress, or alcohol. And don't use an alarm clock or anything else that will awaken you in the morning.

The first time you wake up on Saturday morning—of your own accord—note what time it is, even if you decide to try to squeeze in a little more shut-eye. Do this again Saturday night. By Sunday morning, you should be able to identify what your body naturally requests.

So, for example, if your natural waking time came after seven hours of sleep, then that's what your body is asking for.

During the weekdays, decide when you need to be up and work backward to make sure you're relaxing in bed a half-hour prior to when you need to be asleep. Following the seven-hour example, if you need to be up at 6 a.m., then plan to be in bed at 10:30. Don't eat within three hours of that time, and avoid stimulants such as caffeine, vigorous exercise, excessive stress, or anything else that might cause you to toss and turn and miss your predetermined sleep start.

Once you start getting sufficient, healthy sleep, you won't need an alarm clock to wake up in the morning, and you'll feel alert without needing to drug yourself with stimulants like coffee or cola.

Of course, life doesn't always allow for a steady routine, so occasionally we need help waking up when our schedules change. A quiet alarm clock can nudge you out of a pre-dawn slumber, but if every morning you rely on a blaring alarm—and multiple rounds with the snooze button—you need to seriously reconsider whether you're getting the amount of sleep your body needs.

Cellular Truths

The Vital Role of Sleep in Cellular Repair

Sleep's power to rebuild your body goes well beyond simply providing rest. Sleep triggers the response patterns of hormones that stimulate the cells to repair the damage of a day's activities.

Perhaps the most important is human growth hormone (HGH), which stimulates cell growth by mediating the metabolism of protein, fats, and carbohydrates. HGH also influences weight control by telling fat cells to release the energy in the lipids they are storing and to reduce additional storage.

Your body seems to know when it's appropriate to bring in the maintenance staff, which isn't when you're engaged in normal daily activities such as work and play. Thus, as much as 70 percent of the growth hormone produced in any twenty-four-hour period is secreted while you are sleeping.

The time you schedule for sleep is important. You may enjoy evening activities such as shows and concerts, but your body begins preparing for sleep as soon as the sun goes down, most importantly by secreting melatonin. Secreting growth hormone begins not long after, and more HGH is released during the earlier hours of the night rather than later.

Work Hard to Sleep Hard

We all know how great we feel after a good night's sleep, especially after a long day of hard work or play. It's almost as though we've been given a new lease on life. The connection between the two is no coincidence. Real physical activity—the kind that wears us out—helps us achieve better rest.

What you consider "work," however, may be shortchanging your ability to achieve sweet and satisfying slumber. There's an equation you may remember: Work equals force times distance. So sitting at a desk doesn't count for real work. Your brain is getting tired, but that's about it. Your butt starts to feel paralyzed, your legs are restless, your neck is stiff, and your belly muscles are lax. Desk jobs don't require us to exercise our muscles and joints. Not only are our lungs and heart getting flabby and sluggish, but after a day of this sort of inactivity, we also can't sleep.

The result is that eight hours of sleep from 10 p.m. to 6 a.m. produces a greater level of HGH than would occur during the same amount of sleep from midnight to 8 a.m. Secretion spikes during periods of deep sleep, and those periods more often occur earlier in the night and in the very early morning.

Typically, the rate of production of growth hormone declines as you get older, and that decline can begin as early as when you're in your twenties. The use of artificially produced HGH as therapy is highly controversial, so your best bet is to get your maximal amount of growth hormone the natural way—through adequate amounts of healthy sleep at the right time of night.

By giving our minds over to passively surfing the Internet throughout the day and then remaining ever engaged with technology and machines in the evening, many of us are spending the majority of our time not really working. Inevitably, this is followed by a night in which we're not really resting.

Throwing a Frisbee and chasing your dog around the park—things we would normally define as "play"—are truer examples of "work" than what many of us do each day. That's because when you pile back into your car with that smelly, panting canine, you experience a tangible sense of accomplishment, and you've had a good physical workout—much more so than you would have experienced surfing the web.

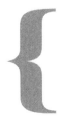

> Many of us are spending the majority of our time not really working . . . followed by a night in which we're not really resting.

Office workers can and should seek out creative outlets that provide good, strenuous labor. I found mine playing indoor soccer and sand volleyball, and I sleep sounder after an evening spent chasing a ball for an hour. The straining of my muscles, coupled with heightened oxygen and blood flow, is what allows my mind to be clear after hard physical work.

Without physical work or play—and yes, sex counts for "play"—cells become so depleted of energy they begin to malfunction.

Sleep quality can also be affected by what happens right before you head to bed. A stressful phone call or stimulating movie or computer game can keep your mind racing at a time when it should be shutting down.

To avoid this, allow yourself time to settle before calling it a day. Just think about how children fall asleep each night. They usually have a bedtime ritual, and so should you. When Andrew was only a few months old, he traveled with Reneé and me for nearly a month. That, combined with evening social events, put him on a crazy schedule—or, I should say, a *lack* of a schedule. Reneé finally put her foot down, and with less travel and a real routine, he went from waking up four to five times per night to sleeping through the night.

Simple Solution:

If you have an office job or an inactive lifestyle, find a physical hobby or activity that allows your body to really work for its rest.

Don't be fooled into thinking a regular sleep schedule is just for kids. Find a regular, evening routine that allows you to slow down, organize, and prepare for the next day. At least one hour before bedtime, turn off distractions that stimulate your mind, such as television, computers, and artificial light. And leave those stressful conversations about work or family problems out of the bedroom, or at least have them a few hours before trying to go to sleep.

A Menu for Healthy Sleep

- Eat three hours or more prior to pillow time. Sleep is for cellular repair, not digesting that 9 p.m. steak dinner. If your digestive system—which involves the largest portion of your body—is working to break down your late dinner or snack, precious energy is being expended rather than stored for the next day's activities. (And don't forget the sleep-depriving heartburn.)
- Limit your caffeine intake. Don't consume more than 200 mg of caffeine—the amount found in about two cups of brewed coffee—per day. If you have more than that, you may experience irritability, heartbeat irregularity, and difficulty falling asleep or sleeping soundly. Commit to gradually cutting back, especially later in the day. Also be aware of caffeine in green teas and soft drinks.
- Keep an accurate count of your alcoholic drinks. Refrain from drinking alcoholic beverages closer than one to one and a half hours before bed.

Libido Boosters

Aside from sleep, the second most important activity that takes place in the master bedroom is sex. Unfortunately, few couples score better in this department than they do with sleep. In a recent survey of more than 12,000 men and women in twenty-seven countries, half of adults reported they weren't fully satisfied with their sex life, and one-third said they were having less sex than they should.[8]

Although there are many reasons why we may not be having enough sex, some of the most common can be addressed by making changes already mentioned in this section.

■ Get some sleep: One of the most common reasons adults give for not having enough sex is just feeling too tired. It confirms what scientists already know: Adopting better sleeping habits can have a positive impact on our libido.

■ Eliminate distractions: Watching television or surfing the Net in bed doesn't just affect the quality of our sleep. Couples also report that it creates a serious diversion when it comes to sex. Why not get rid of the TV and create your own entertainment instead?

■ Declutter and destress: A getaway to a five-star hotel makes many of us feel more amorous. Why? For most, it's what is *not* in the hotel room that puts us in the mood. Gone are the piles of laundry, stacks of bills, and stressful conversations that so often await us in our master bedrooms at home. So keep your bedroom clean and comfortable. Make it a place of refuge, where nagging tasks and stressful arguments aren't allowed.

■ Work those muscles: Physical exertion—whether walking two miles or skiing a tough run—can give a big boost to our sexual satisfaction, and it's not because of slimmer thighs or killer abs. That feeling of exhilaration we get after a tough workout is actually a release of endorphins in the brain, the same chemicals that have been linked to the release of hormones that increase the sex drive.

In the classic children's book *Where the Wild Things Are* by Maurice Sendak, Max, the book's young hero, falls asleep one evening and journeys to the land of the "Wild Things," scary monsters that Max must conquer.

Things that go bump in the night and imaginary ghouls may be part of our childhood books, but as this section has revealed, the scary stuff isn't what might be hiding under the bed—it's what we have lurking in our mattresses, hiding in the sheets, or hovering over our pillows.

Even if we're successful in getting plenty of shut-eye, we may still be subjecting our bodies to unseen dangers that take a cumulative toll over time. Many of us are sleeping with the enemy—air that is heavy with fumes, sheets that spew chemical fragrance, and electronic devices that generate EMFs in every corner of the bedroom.

While evaluating our sleeping and lovemaking environment, cleaning out the clutter is a great place to start. And give serious thought to what you can do to create sleep with as few distractions as possible. There are many things you can do to improve your sleeping environment and to maximize your body's ability to heal during those critical hours of cellular repair.

Even Up the Score

You likely garnered some danger points in your chapter quizzes, but don't get discouraged. Below you'll find a wide range of changes you can make to improve your bedroom—each assigned its own point value. Your goal should be to make enough small changes to get your "Bedroom Health" score above zero.

Be sure to get your Web code in the back of this book and join us online at www.myhealthyhome.com to get even more solutions, update your scores, and get involved in making a positive difference in the health of your home. You may even win some prizes for your efforts!

SOLUTIONS SUMMARY

What Simple Solutions will you add to your Bedroom?

	Scores
1. I will: (Select one)	
☐ Switch to natural fabrics for pajamas (4 pts) and/or sheets (4 pts)	
☐ Switch to organic cotton pajamas (6 pts) and/or sheets (6 pts)	
2. I will: (Select all that apply)	
☐ Use a green, nontoxic laundry detergent (6 pts)	
☐ Switch to a fragrance-free, mainstream brand of detergent (3 pts)	
☐ Eliminate my use of dryer sheets (6 pts)	
3. I will: (Select all that apply)	
☐ Eliminate dry cleaning altogether (12 pts)	
☐ Reduce use of "perc" dry cleaning to real necessities (4 pts)	
☐ Air out dry cleaning before bringing it into the house (2 pts)	
☐ Switch to a green dry cleaner (8 pts)	
☐ Wear an undershirt made of natural fibers beneath dry-cleaned clothing (2 pts)	
4. I will: (Select all that apply)	
☐ Eliminate all constrictive clothing (10 pts)	
☐ Remove tight clothing, like bras and shirts with snug collars, when at home (4 pts)	
☐ Honestly assess my wardrobe and give away clothing items that are too tight (8 pts)	
5. I will: (Select all that apply)	
☐ Switch to an organic or natural rubber mattress (15 pts)	
☐ Air out my mattress whenever laundering the bedding (3 pts)	
☐ Use a natural rubber or organic wool mattress cover (6 pts)	

6. I will: (Select all that apply)

☐ Move electronics away from bed (3 pts for each item moved at least four feet)

☐ Regularly unplug appliances and gadgets when not in use (5 pts)

☐ Eliminate use of electric blanket or unplug it before getting into bed (10 pts)

7. I will: (Select one)

☐ Reduce bedroom light to zero while sleeping (7 pts)

☐ Move or replace electronics in the bedroom that feature white or blue light (4 pts)

8. I will: (Select all that apply)

☐ Take a melatonin supplement before bed to support the body's natural sleep processes (4 pts)

☐ Heat or cool the room enough to ensure I don't wake up too hot or cold (3 pts)

9. I will: (Select all that apply)

☐ Perform the weekend sleeping experiment on pages 55–56 to see how much rest my body really needs (4 pts)

☐ Set a reasonable bedtime and stick to it—during weekdays and weekends (6 pts)

☐ Adjust sleep schedule to get to bed before 10:30 p.m. to maximize melatonin and HGH production (6 pts)

10. I will: (Select all that apply)

☐ Get physical activity—"real work" as referenced in the text—each day (5 pts)

☐ Eliminate caffeine or food three hours prior to bedtime (5 pts)

☐ Create a winding down routine and follow it every night (3 pts)

☐ Avoid stimulation like video games and television at least thirty minutes prior to bedtime (3 pts)

Your Simple Solutions positive score: ☐

Your "Rub" danger score: | - |

Your "Electric" danger score: | - |

Your "Sleep" danger score: | - |

Your Bedroom Health total: ☐

Are you making a positive difference? Keep working at making one or two Simple Solutions at a time until your score is well into the positive. It doesn't have to be arduous—just be willing to make regular "baby steps." Many small changes over a lifetime will add up to better health.

You can track your quiz scores and solution points on *The Healthy Home* Web site at www.myhealthyhome.com.

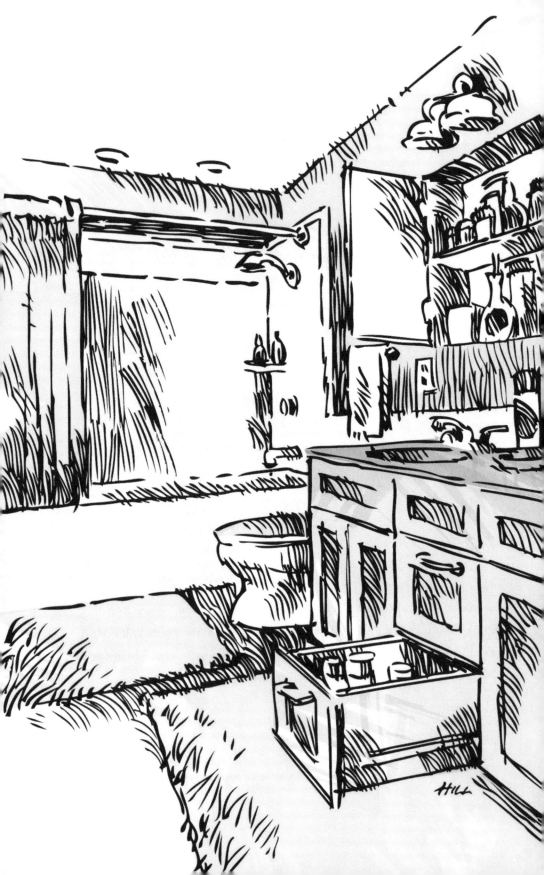

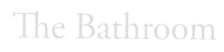

3

The Bathroom

Bleary-eyed, we stumble each day into the bathroom, largely unaware of our early morning surroundings. We feel safe in our home sweet homes, yet our bathrooms might as well have the skull and crossbones symbol displayed on the door.

Many bathrooms have more toxic chemicals than the garage. The more bottles and tubes there are sitting on the counter, lined up in the medicine cabinet, packed in drawers, and stashed in the shower, the more poison you are likely accumulating in your body. This section will reveal what ought to trigger the greatest concern, what to avoid, and what simple solutions can be easily employed to protect your health without sacrificing the universal goal of looking your best.

Having finished the tour of Dave's newly renovated master bedroom, Dr. Wentz makes his way into the master bathroom. Stylishly designed, it boasts beautiful natural stone, contemporary lines, warm earth colors, thick towels, and a spa-like shower—the ultimate escape from even the most stressful day.

How could there possibly be any danger in there?

Dave: Dad, maybe you shouldn't go in there.

Dr. Wentz: *[Smiling as he opens the cabinet next to the sink.]* The bathroom has a tremendous impact on our health. It rivals the kitchen in its importance for determining our quality of life.

Donna: How so?

Dave: When we think about changing habits to improve our health, we usually think about changes in our eating habits. But because the bathroom is small, often poorly ventilated, and heavily contaminated, it's one of the most dangerous places in the house for heavy metals, endocrine disruptors, and VOCs—and most dangerous for me if I don't get my dad out of there before he starts tossing my wife's hair products.

Dr. Wentz: *[Holding up a bottle of hair spray for closer inspection.]* Actually, I'm pretty impressed. So far I've only found seven things for you to throw out.

Donna: Because the dates have expired?

Dave: No, it's not that. The problem is that most people underestimate the chemicals present in their personal-care products.

Dr. Wentz: I always urge people to look at their product labels. They'll likely find thirty or forty ingredients, most of which are unrecognizable to a layperson. But we spread them all over our face, hair, and skin without so much as a question to their safety. What's this? Dave, you aren't using antiperspirant are you?

Dave: Well, I find it necessary at times, as you might imagine. However, notice that deodorant right next to it? I use that on weekends or other times when I don't have to worry if people see me sweat.

Dr. Wentz: Hmm, you know how I feel about aluminum in personal-care products. *[Opening a drawer.]* I see your toothpaste is fluoride-free. Well done. But I also see mouthwash . . .

Dave: My mistake. That's been sitting there for a few years. I've long since stopped using mouthwash. For some reason I think we're all bad about throwing unused things out.

Dr. Wentz: Especially with things we perceive as valuable. Even though it's a very dangerous practice, people don't dispose of unused prescription drugs for that reason. They feel as if an antibiotic or painkiller may be of use sometime down the road. But it looks like acetaminophen is your most dangerous one here.

Chapter 4
Let's Get Personal

When considering the dangers that might lurk in the bathroom, the first ones that come to mind are tile cleansers, toilet scrub, bleaches, and other cleaning products that leave toxic smells hanging in the air, choking us until we can get the job done and escape.

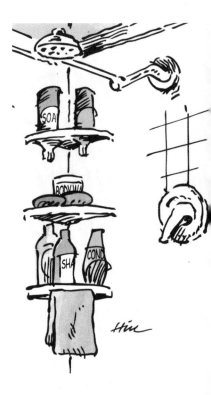

But cleaners are only a small part of a frightening list of chemicals we need to address. Many more—found in personal-care products like lotion, antiperspirant, cleansers, makeup, and hairspray—can do just as much damage. Perhaps more so because we don't take precautions like we do when we use bleach or drain cleaner.

In fact, we let these dangerous products sit on our skin all day long.

How Toxic Is Your Home?

Scores

1. How much cologne or perfume do you typically wear? (Select one)

   ☐ None (0 pts)   ☐ A full spritz (4 pts)
   ☐ Just a dab (2 pts)   ☐ A big splash or multiple spritzes (6 pts)

2. How many aerosol products do you use? Consider antiperspirants, hairsprays, and so forth. (7 pts each)

3. Do you use an antiperspirant deodorant? (Check your product label if you're not sure.)
   Yes_____ (7 pts)

4. How many personal-care products do you use each day? Consider products listed above as well as cosmetic, shaving, and skin-care products. (2 pts each)

Your "Personal" danger score

1–8	9–16	17–24	25+
Natural beauty	Time to refresh	Some ugly habits	Chemical complexion

Lotions and Potions

Skin is an intricate mesh that provides a partial barrier against environmental elements—good and bad—but it lets in far more than we realize. Consider all of the drugs and therapies being made available in skin patches to treat such things as motion sickness, nicotine withdrawal, heart disease, and pain. These patches deliver drugs through the skin and directly to the bloodstream.

Although the skin is good at absorbing things, it also excretes toxins from the body through our pores. Given the vital roles it performs, protecting our skin is as important as watching what we eat and drink.

My father often says, "If you aren't willing to eat something, you shouldn't put it on your skin." And he's correct. If we're afraid to spray that antiperspirant on our tongue or squeeze a glob of that eye cream in our mouth, we shouldn't put it on our skin. After all, the same toxic chemicals we refuse to ingest are still entering our bodies and circulating to our cells. When our company launched a skin-care line free of paraben preservatives, Dr. Wentz stood on stage in front of thousands of people and squeezed a small portion of lotion on his tongue to prove his point. Skin-care products should be made from natural and healthy ingredients—they may not taste good, but they shouldn't do us harm.

A Toxic Cover-up?

Who doesn't imagine a firmer, less-wrinkled tomorrow as promised by sexy advertisements and airbrushed photos? We might even consider ourselves addicted to the pursuit of beauty. In our culture, beauty equals success, and we each hope for the miracle of vibrant skin, luscious lips, and shiny hair.

Men and women alike enjoy trying new products and openly confess to being gullible when manufacturers release new potions that claim to halt aging or hair products that promise thicker textures. They keep life interesting and fun, and we're game for anything that promises to slow the clock.

When taking the quiz at the beginning of this chapter, you may have been surprised at just how many different personal-care products you use on a daily basis. You're not alone. A 2004 survey of 2,300 American men and women found that the average adult uses nine products—containing around 126 individual ingredients—every day.[1]

Nine or more products every day? That's a lot of fragrances, preservatives, and other chemicals coating the body's largest organ.

We assume these products must be safe or else they wouldn't be on store shelves. If your bathroom cabinet resembles most others, however, you have a chemical stockpile that should make your hair turn gray. Just read down the list of ingredients on your makeup removers, body washes, shaving foams, shampoos, conditioners, antiperspirants, moisturizers, lipsticks, foundations, powders, liquid liners, pencils, hair gels, mousses, sprays, toothpastes, rinses, whiteners, perfumes, nail polishes, sunscreens, spray-on tanners, bug sprays— even toilet paper, tampons, and bandages have chemicals added.

Do you ever wonder just how many chemicals are being absorbed through the skin and into the body when we use these items? You don't have to wonder. A recent study found more than two hundred chemicals present just in the umbilical cord blood of newborns.[2] Once our infants leave the relative safety of the womb, how many more sweet-smelling chemical compounds do we deliberately subject them to?

> Nine or more products every day? That's a lot of fragrances, preservatives, and other chemicals coating the body's largest organ.

Keep in mind that personal-care products such as those listed above are typically only tested on adults. An estimated 10,500 different chemicals are used in cosmetics, skin-care treatments, and other personal products. Some of these chemicals are nitrosamines, lead and other heavy metals, parabens, phthalates, hydroquinone, and 1,4-dioxane—all very bad stuff.[3]

In fact, 1,4-dioxane is a probable carcinogen found in almost a quarter of all cosmetic products—not as an ingredient, but as a contaminant.[4]

How Much Poison Is Too Much?

Knowing that these products have such dangerous ingredients, the next logical question is: How can it be legal to sell toxic products to unsuspecting customers?

The government has come up with the term "maximum safe levels" to tell you how much of a toxic ingredient your body should be able to withstand. This is the government's blanket way of saying that a scientist has informed them that, based on animal studies, five parts per million of a particular ingredient doesn't cause health problems that they can detect. At higher levels, however, this same ingredient may show signs of causing anything from hives to cancer.

That such studies have been done may sound reassuring, but the groups typically performing toxicity studies on skin-care ingredients are the manufacturers themselves who want their products to make it to market. Yet when it comes to clinical studies, I could design one that shows cyanide was safe in mice. All I would have to do is evaluate the mice two seconds after the cyanide was administered and conclude that they were fine. Yet if I waited a minute to record the data, all the mice would be dead.

Although this example may seem a little silly, it shows the very real dangers of performing short-term studies on ingredients that might have long-term, cumulative effects. Cancer and other degenerative diseases take years to develop. On top of that, there are simply too many variables to look for in any single study. Yet as far as some manufacturers are concerned, safety is secondary. New chemicals are considered safe until *proven* dangerous, and for many consumers, by then it may be too late.

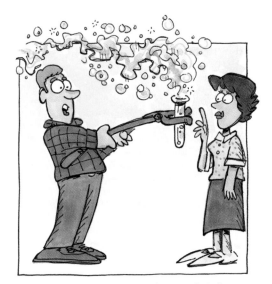

"It's poisonous, so just take a small sip."

Personal-care industry experts often claim that the incriminating studies—such as those showing a risk of cancer—are unrealistic. After all, they say, the studies may have used ten times the "normal dose" or "maximum safe level" of an ingredient recommended in the use of that product. But what if you were to use ten products with the maximum safe level of the same ingredient, or use them for ten times longer than the study ran? Did someone actually decide that one-tenth of the poison that kills you is safe? If I cannot find pancreatic cancer in subjects who smoke one cigarette per day, can I then conclude that one cigarette per day is safe?

For that matter, are those who are conducting the studies assuming that you have a perfectly healthy immune system, liver, kidneys, and lymph drainage as well as excellent air quality and drinking water? Quite the opposite—it's more realistic to assume that your body is battling a hundred other cellular attacks at any given time.

Although we can't go into *all* of the hidden dangers found in personal-care products, we can delve into some of the most common ones and discover ways to avoid them.

"Preserving" Beauty

Manufacturers know what consumers want, and they deliver. They know that one of the major turnoffs for consumers is opening a jar of cosmetics and finding that it has become moldy. At the same time, they want to be able to ship their products long distances and store them in warehouses for months in order to make distribution efficient. That's why nearly all cosmetics contain preservative chemicals.

Preservatives, by their very nature, are designed to be cytotoxic—in other words, they kill cells. Specifically, they work by preventing the growth of bacteria and fungi—mainly *Candida albicans, Pseudomonas aeruginosa, Escherichia coli, Aspergillus niger,* and *Staphylococcus aureus*—that can potentially cause infections on the skin and in the body.

> Preservatives, by their very nature, are designed to be cytotoxic—in other words, they kill cells.

The problem is that human skin is also made of cells, so preservatives—even if used in small quantities—present a risk to the integrity of the skin cells. When absorbed into the bloodstream, preservatives also become a hazard to the rest of the body. For this reason, preservative levels are restricted to a small percentage of the total formula.

Just a little bit of poison.

We're exposed to an astonishing number of chemicals every day, and we rarely think about the cumulative effects they might have on our health. When we stop to reflect on a particular product's ingredient panel, most of us shrug and assume, "It must be safe. They wouldn't sell it if it wasn't."

The things you love most about your products are often created by adding particular ingredients "at maximum safe levels." But what are those levels for you and your body when you:

- Wash your face, tone, and exfoliate?
- Apply a masque, moisturize, and use eye cream?
- Add foundation, mascara, lipstick, eye liner, and blush?
- Use shampoo, conditioner, and hairspray?

Get the point?

So let's say the government has concluded that they can't find health problems with a preservative used in skin-care products as long as the amount of the preservative doesn't exceed a certain level. This is good news to the face cream manufacturer—we'll call it Company A—that wants to create a product that has the longest shelf life possible while killing the bugs that tend to grow in such a moist, nutrient-rich environment. Company A, therefore, puts the maximum amount of preservative the government will allow in its product, and everyone is happy.

Of course, Company B has the same plan for its eye cream that effectively prevents wrinkles. And Company C needs to be competitive with its masque product. To keep their products from going bad before they can sell them, Companies B and C also add the maximum amount of the very same preservative to each of *their* products.

All of these products are deemed safe and compliant according to government regulations that assume you must be living in a vacuum.

Unfortunately, when you add up the face cream, eye cream, and masque, your face is receiving *three times* the

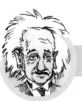

Ask the Scientist

"Dr. Wentz, why are parabens of particular concern to you?"

Parabens are toxic chemical preservatives and are the most common of all ingredients found in skin-care products. It is estimated that women are exposed to as much as 50 mg of parabens every day from cosmetics and personal-care products alone.[5] Parabens exhibit estrogenic activity and are suspected of being carcinogenic.

Current evidence shows parabens to be weak hormone mimics, but among adolescent girls who are undergoing an onslaught of hormonal activity as they develop into mature women, it doesn't take much to upset the normal transformation from child into adult.

There are some disturbing changes occurring in our young women today. Girls begin developing breasts one to two years earlier than they did forty years ago. About half of all U.S. girls show signs of breast development by their tenth birthday, with 14 percent attaining breast buds between their eighth and ninth birthdays. They are losing a significant portion of their childhood.

maximum safe level of that particular preservative when all three products become part of your daily regimen—and that doesn't even take into account makeup and hair-care products.

These toxins will sit on your face and skin all day long. You may even reapply them throughout the day. By using all of these products, you inevitably damage the very cells you're trying to keep looking vibrant and healthy.

What about your shaving cream, cologne, antiperspirant, shower gel, shampoo, and sunscreen? If you're putting the maximum safe level on your body in six different products, you now have *six times* the safe dose of those chemicals headed to your bloodstream.

On average, adult women use twelve personal care products per day, whereas teenage girls use an average of seventeen cosmetic and personal care products daily.[6] That means they are applying *hundreds* of chemicals—many of them of unknown effect or safety—to their skin and hair. One study of teenagers found an average of thirteen different hormone-altering chemicals in their bodies.[7]

With this level of toxic exposure, it can't be a surprise that young women today are demonstrating abnormal, premature sexual development.

All Grown Up

TRUE OR FALSE? **Some preservatives contained in beauty products can accumulate and alter sexual development in children.**

True.

We worry and fuss about our kids eating well and getting enough rest and exercise, and then we give our daughters toxic perfumes or colognes, makeup, body lotions, and spritzers that they wear all day. As a result, while they are dreaming of being all grown up, our young girls are absorbing toxins and breathing in chemical fumes that, according to the government, aren't dangerous enough to kill them. Yet these chemicals are proven to impact hormone systems severely enough to fast-forward ten-year-olds into sexual maturity.

We're finally seeing concern grow over the cumulative effect of parabens and phthalates contained in preservatives, and it's about time. What do you envision for your adolescent daughter, granddaughter, or niece? Teen idols aren't the only bad influence on them. Industry regulators say parabens are safe, but scientists examining their effects in lab

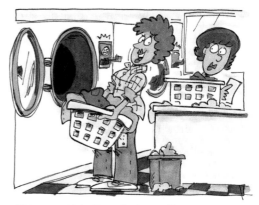

"It turns out I don't need estrogen therapy anymore. I just wash my clothes with detergents with phthalates and use lots of paraben-filled lotion."

animals and marine life find that these toxins are hormone disruptors.

For now, it's best to play it safe. Preteen girls shouldn't be allowed to use makeup or other adult cosmetic products, no matter how much they beg. And it's best to encourage teenagers to keep the use of all of their personal-care products to a minimum.

Formaldehyde-release Agents

Formaldehyde—which you may remember from your high school biology class as the strong-smelling solution used to preserve dead frogs—is toxic to cells and can cause cancer. But it's also highly effective at killing microbes, which makes it an effective preservative.

To get around some of the health risks posed by formaldehyde, manufacturers have created a class of compounds known as formaldehyde-release agents, so called because they release small amounts of formaldehyde into products to keep them free of contaminants. Fortunately, many people have allergic reactions to these smaller doses of the potent solution, and thus know to avoid these products.

Simple Solution:
Cut down on toxic preservatives like parabens, phthalates, and formaldehyde by first replacing products that sit on your skin all day—like a moisturizer—with more natural, preservative-free alternatives.

Unfortunately, the rest of us don't have visible reactions that will warn us to avoid these products. So we're left to find out the hard way just how much formaldehyde our bodies can combat. Japan as a country has taken a proactive stance against this potentially dangerous compound, having banned formaldehyde completely from personal-care products.

See for yourself how many of your own products contain formaldehyde-release agents. They'll likely be listed on your labels as: [8]

- Quaternium 15
- 2-bromo-2-nitropropane-1,3-diol
- Diazolidinyl urea
- Imidazolidinyl urea
- DMDM Hydantoin

"Look Older with Prolonged Use!"

It's not much of a tagline for a skin-care product.

Yet many "anti-aging" products contain chemicals that are cytotoxic to your skin cells, so they actually damage them over time. It's quite a business model, really, when you can convince someone that a product will make them look better and at the same time damage the skin so they will need to buy more products.

Using makeup or temporary skin-care fixes to hide damaged skin is like painting over rust. Unless you first remove the rust itself, the damage underneath will continue to undermine the beauty on the surface. If you're worried about hiding dry skin, blemishes, acne, and such, you should first address your diet, sun protection, immune system, and general health to help with the underlying problem.

Simple Solution:
Focus on eliminating the *cause* of your skin problems—not on covering up the symptoms.

For instance, consider whether you are drinking enough water to hydrate the skin cells, consuming enough essential fatty acids, vitamins, minerals, and other nutrients to properly nourish the skin cells, and keeping chemicals and pollutants off your skin.

Scentsibility

Have you ever entered an elevator and found that someone's cologne or perfume was so strong that you could barely breathe? I'll bet you money the person wearing the scent couldn't smell it at all. Our bodies have an amazing ability to become desensitized to familiar scents and stop sending the warning signal to our brains. This phenomenon is especially noticeable when you visit a farm, where the odor of manure is overwhelming at first, and barely noticeable a few hours later.

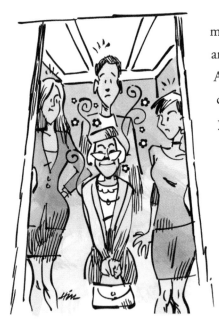

As we learned in chapter 1, fragrances in most laundry and personal-care products today are created in laboratories, not fields of flowers. Although finding a fragrance-free detergent can be fairly simple, avoiding fragrances in your skin-care products is a more difficult task. Moisturizers, creams, and scrubs often contain smelly lipids, humectants, and other ingredients you really wouldn't want to rub on your face every morning. For this reason, some sort of fragrance—or a masking ingredient that renders the product "unscented"—is typically added to skin-care products to make those ingredients more pleasant to our finicky noses.

Natural oils can be used as a fragrance, but often they aren't stable and quickly deteriorate. That's why you'll find artificial fragrances or masking ingredients in just about every skin-care product today—especially the ones with a longer shelf life.

Although fragrance may be necessary in more complex skin-care products, we can reduce our exposure in this area by switching to less heavily scented products. After all, do we really need five or six fragrances competing with each other?

- A moisturizer that smells like lavender
- An antiperspirant scented like peach
- Shampoo and conditioner that smell like honey
- A shower gel scented like pear

Many of us begin to smell like a fruit salad with all those chemicals wafting around our body. By buying lightly scented or *genuinely* unscented products for the majority of our personal-care regimen and allowing ourselves just one or two products with a stronger fragrance, we'll be cutting down on chemicals—and sparing those who share our space.

An Aerosol Cloud

Now we know that we have toxic ingredients in our skin-care products and that they are primarily absorbed through our skin. We also know they are slowly off-gassing into the air around us because we can smell them. So why on earth would we make matters worse by using an aerosol spray product that spews half of the product directly into the air?

Simple Solution:
Avoid aerosol products that have nonspray alternatives. If you must use aerosols, open a window and run your bathroom fan.

These chemicals are absorbed far more quickly through our mouths and our lungs. Plus, an aerosol spray will subject our family members to whatever toxins we've just applied. Get that toxic cloud out of your bathroom—and out of your lungs.

Then What Is Safe?

As consumers become more informed about what's in the products they're using, manufacturers are growing ever-more clever in *how* they present ingredients. "Natural" formulas are often created by adding natural-sounding ingredients such as honey or herbs or aloe without actually removing the unhealthy, unnatural ingredients.

Take the time to read product labels; you'll find that there are a lot of good nontoxic alternatives on the market that avoid using the chemicals we've just discussed. As a starting point, steer clear of products that have the following ingredients listed on their labels, especially if the products will be used by children:

- Parabens (methyl, propyl, butyl, and ethyl)
- Mercury (thimerosal)
- Lead acetate
- Diethanolamine (DEA)
- Synthetic color pigments
- Propylene glycol (PG)
- Coal tar
- Toluene
- Phenylenediamine (PPD)
- Petrolatum

Also cut way back on all product use if you are pregnant because your unborn baby will be subjected to the same products you use on yourself.

Simple Solution:
Wash products off your face as soon as you get home instead of waiting until bedtime. A few additional chemical-free hours each day could add up to more than six years over a lifetime.

And while you're looking through your personal-care products, be sure to toss all of those with expired dates.

Focus first and foremost on products that sit on your skin all day and night before you tackle those that you rinse off.

If you're feeling overwhelmed by all this, remember that making even a few small changes will help lessen the cumulative effects of toxic substances on your skin. Just think, if you stop using just two of ten products you use every day, you're reducing your burden by 20 percent. Multiply that by 365 days of the year, year after year. That small change will have a huge cumulative impact on your long-term health. Be aware of potential dangers and choose alternatives where possible—it could make a long-term difference as you choose between cancer-free and wrinkle-free.

Which is more important to you?

> If you stop using just two of ten products you use every day, you're reducing your burden by 20 percent. Multiply that by 365 days of the year, year after year.

The Stink about Antiperspirants

Junior high school is a strange chapter in life—indeed, many embarrassing memories of early adolescence still haunt me today. Somehow we managed to survive the cafeteria food, awkward first attempts at dating, and smelly feet in gym class. But just a couple of decades later, most adults retain a few of the social fears that drag them back to that paralyzing feeling of insecurity.

One of those fears was looking or smelling sweaty. As students, we would point and laugh if someone raised his or her arms and had sweaty pits. So we coated on the antiperspirant as thick as we could. Most of us still do it today. The trouble is that in doing so, we're inhibiting one of the body's natural processes.

Aluminum: A Deadly Ingredient

Although antiperspirants and deodorants are often mixed together to create a single product and they share the same shelves at the pharmacy or superstore, they are two very different consumables that work in markedly different ways.

Antiperspirants operate on the principle that if you don't sweat, you don't smell. How do you keep from sweating? Easy: You plug and disable your sweat glands and pores. Nearly all antiperspirants accomplish this task by using aluminum compounds—usually aluminum chlorohydrate or aluminum zirconium.

Deodorants, however, don't keep you from sweating. Instead, the alcohol or other chemicals kill some bacteria, and the burst of fragrance covers the odors caused by any bacteria that remain. Nonantiperspirant deodorant products do not typically contain aluminum compounds.

As a corporate executive, I've spoken at numerous events—with thousands of people in the audience—typically followed by an hour or more of greeting and hand shaking.

My nerves during the first few years of public speaking caused me to exhibit what I feared was social suicide—sweaty palms. Rather than risk the embarrassment of offering up a clammy hand to a colleague or business associate, I would rub clinical-strength antiperspirant into my hands for several nights leading up to an event, despite the

Toxic Effects of Aluminum on the Cell

Although aluminum is the third most abundant element on earth, it serves no useful function in the human body. Its presence results only in toxicity and malfunction in cell structures and biological systems.

The target organs for aluminum toxicity are primarily the lungs, bones, and the central nervous system. Animal studies show that aluminum in the nervous system results in altered expression of cytoskeletal genes and damage to structural proteins in brain cells, including the formation of phosphate-rich protein filaments. These proteins are seen in several neurological diseases, including dementia, multiple sclerosis, and Alzheimer's disease.

In general, the greatest accumulation of aluminum is in large, long-lived, nondividing cells such as neurons. Aluminum binds irreversibly to molecules within the nucleus, cross-linking the DNA and blocking DNA replication. If the cross-linking isn't repaired, the result is replication arrest and cell death.

Aluminum accumulates within the cell in the lysosomes, nucleus, and chromatin, where it reacts strongly with many important molecules. Aluminum competes molecularly

fact that my skin would burn for hours after the application. Even worse, I was making a conscious trade-off between social embarrassment and the threat of health problems that would appear down the road.

Even then I knew there were possible links between aluminum compounds and everything from breast cancer and kidney failure to Alzheimer's and Parkinson's disease. Fortunately, I've moved past my phobia of public speaking and have given up this bizarre application of antiperspirant.

However, many people still persist in using antiperspirants and running the risk of serious problems later in life. Our social fears continue to take precedence over our fundamental survival instinct.

with minerals important to biological systems—especially magnesium but also calcium. Aluminum competes with iron for transferrin, and thus is distributed to every organ and tissue in the body.

Finally, aluminum can induce oxidative damage, impairing function in vital cell membranes. Aluminum-induced oxidative damage to the lipid-rich myelin sheath—which makes nerve function possible—has been linked to Parkinson's and amyotrophic lateral sclerosis (ALS).[9]

Aluminum Toxicity

The concern with aluminum is, again, a cumulative one. The threat that aluminum poses to our health comes from the fact that it is used in so many products—literally thousands, from stepladders to antiperspirants.

In fact, over-the-counter medications can be one of the most frequent sources of personal contact with aluminum.

- Users of buffered aspirin—such as people with arthritis—might take in up to 500 mg of aluminum each day.
- A typical dose of aluminum-containing antacids can contain as much as 400 mg, and an entire day's use can supply 800–5,000 mg of aluminum.

- Digestive aides such as diarrhea and hemorrhoid remedies can also contain aluminum.
- Food cooked or stored in aluminum pots and aluminum foil can be another source, and aluminum salts are used as additives in cake mixes, frozen dough, pancake mixes, self-rising flours, processed cheese, and cheese foods.

Although there's no known need for aluminum in the human body—or in any animal, as far as we know—aluminum can be found in most animal and plant tissue. Aluminum causes problems in the body largely by competing with several other elements with similar characteristics. If you are deficient in such minerals as magnesium, calcium, or iron, then aluminum is always there to take their place inside your cells. Compare it to building a steel bridge and having a worker add aluminum beams whenever steel isn't available. Your bridge will have many weak spots that don't function properly and will likely collapse.

Just as your cells will collapse.

Although the body tries to excrete most of the aluminum it takes in, any excess is deposited in various tissues including bone, brain, liver, heart, spleen, and muscle. In certain tissues with relatively low turnover—such as the brain—aluminum is difficult to remove once it's in place, resulting in long-term damage.

The bottom line is to know the dangers of aluminum toxicity and weigh the risks. Keep in mind that even though Americans may be annoyed by perspiration, the body has designed this method of cooling and daily cleansing. Using a deodorant that doesn't contain antiperspirant is a good option, especially at times when you know you won't be sweating as much.

An undershirt can also help hide underarm perspiration.

Simple Solution:

Don't use antiperspirant during cooler months or on weekends when it doesn't matter if you sweat a little.

Of course, you may possess overactive sweat glands or live in a humid climate and, thus, may decide that year-round antiperspirant is a must. If so, then you need to tackle aluminum from another angle.

Simple Solution:

If you do wear antiperspirant, wash it off in the evening. You don't need it while you're asleep.

You can avoid other sources of aluminum, such as antacids. Also, consider a detox regimen that will help support your body's ability to cleanse that aluminum, especially getting it out of your brain. Some natural ways to detox include ingesting apple pectin, lemon juice, kelp, or turmeric or taking an old-fashioned Epsom-salt bath.

And when you can, dare to sweat a little.

For more information on detoxification, go to www.myhealthyhome.com/detox.

Chapter 5
Bright, White, and Pearly

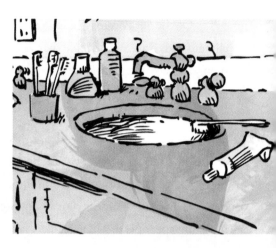

How many elevators have been cleared and budding romances killed by the presence of bad breath? The numbers must be in the millions— on commercials, at least.

Oh, and the agony of teeth that aren't pearly white.

A stroll down the dental aisle at the supermarket or pharmacy can seem overwhelming with its myriad choices: ultra-whitening, sensitivity soothing, breath enhancing, cavity fighting, and tartar preventing. It all sounds so refreshing . . . right?

Taking care of our teeth and gums is a surprisingly important part of total body wellness, yet many of us unknowingly introduce toxins directly into our mouths in a quest to achieve a winning, "healthy looking" smile.

QUIZ

How Toxic Is Your Home?   Scores

1. Do you use fluoride toothpaste? Yes_____ (8 pts)

2. Take stock of your teeth. How many silver-colored fillings do you have in your mouth? (10 pts each)

3. If you don't have silver fillings, enter zero for this question. If you do have silver fillings, which of the following are regular habits for you? (Select all that apply.)
   ☐ Chewing gum (4 pts)   ☐ Chewing ice (3 pts)
   ☐ Drinking hot drinks (coffee, tea, etc.) (4 pts)

4. Which do you use to reduce bad breath? (Select all that apply)
   ☐ Gum (6 pts)   ☐ Mouthwash (4 pts)   ☐ Tongue Scraper (0 pts)

Your "Pearly" danger score

1–12	13–24	25–36	37+
Mile-wide grin	Straight-faced	Grimace	Scowl

Toxic Toothpaste

"Keep out of reach of children under 6 years of age. If more than used for brushing is accidentally swallowed, get medical help or contact a poison control center right away."

You've held these words in your hand once or twice a day for more than a decade. It's a required warning that appears on every tube of fluoridated toothpaste manufactured in the United States. The FDA began requiring this warning in the late 90s when it became clear that small children could be seriously injured—or even killed—by fluoride poisoning.

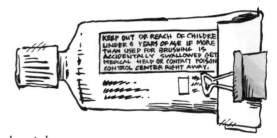

Wait a minute—

Swallowing fluoride toothpaste can be fatal?

It's true, yet many local governments in the United States have passed legislation requiring the fluoridation of public water supplies.

Ironically, ingesting too much fluoride—whether through toothpaste, fluoridated water, or a combination of sources—can actually damage the tooth enamel in young children. The condition, known as enamel fluorosis, can cause a chalky or brown discoloration and pitting of the enamel. The very reason for subjecting ourselves (and our children) to fluoride is ostensibly for the purpose of engendering strong teeth, yet it can have the very opposite effect!

Could we possibly have been lied to? Or should I be more politically correct and say we're "misinformed"?

Absolutely.

Essentially, fluoride is industrial waste that has been remarkably repackaged and effectively marketed over the years for topical products like toothpaste as well as mass treatment of our water supplies.

We can smile easy, though, knowing that we don't have to choose between brushing with poison and having bright, healthy teeth. First, the physical action of the toothbrush is what *really* cleans our teeth, not the toothpaste. And there are excellent fluoride-free toothpastes—available in health stores, at larger grocery chains, and online—that create the minty, foaming sensation we've come to expect while brushing.

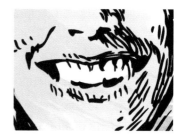

Simple Solution:
Take a daily calcium, magnesium, and vitamin D supplement to help keep your teeth healthy.

Twice-daily brushing, tongue-scraping, and flossing, along with regular dental checkups are all we need to maintain a beautiful smile.

And if you refuse to give up fluoride toothpaste, apply the smallest amount possible to your brush and closely supervise young children to prevent swallowing.

Minty Fresh?

TRUE OR FALSE? Most mouthwashes contain ingredients, such as formaldehyde, that can be harmful if swallowed.

True.

A little soap may have broken you of your cussing habit back when your mom washed out your mouth, but some of the mouthwashes on the market today might be a good reason to curse up a blue streak.

As with the other products we're putting on our skin, we cannot assume that dental products are safe just because they're manufactured for use in our mouths. The same germ killers—phenol, cresol, and ethanol—that are used in bathroom disinfectants are also formulated, though in lower concentrations, in a product designed for use in the mouth. These ingredients could be swallowed and *will* be absorbed through your mouth's soft tissue. Other ingredients in mouthwash include formaldehyde and ammonia. Yet this should come as no surprise. Why else would the label warn against swallowing?

How stupid can it get?

We know which foods bring on the bad breath. Garlic and onions, for example, get absorbed in the bloodstream and are exhaled through the lungs, and this process can continue for days after you've eaten them. Tobacco use, of course, causes bad breath, but so can dry mouth because saliva helps to clean the mouth. And when bacteria break down food particles in between your teeth, foul-smelling breath can also result.

Daily brushing, flossing, and drinking plenty of pure water should keep gums healthy and prevent bad breath. But if you have lingering halitosis, you may want to try the regular use of a tongue scraper, which can be found on the dental aisle at most drug stores. This simple tool will do far more than a chemical mouthwash to help solve bad breath.

Simple Solution:
Consider rinsing with water flavored with an extract such as peppermint, anise, or cinnamon.

A Mouth Full of Poison

Lean close to the mirror and open wide.

Take a close look at your teeth. What do you see?

This is one time you don't want to see a silver lining. Those silver-colored fillings are made of mercury. Every time you chew or drink hot liquids with metal fillings in your teeth, vapors of mercury—the most toxic nonradioactive metal on planet earth—are being released and absorbed in your mouth.

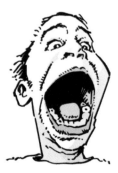

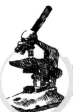

Cellular Truths

Mercury is the only metal that's liquid in its elemental state. Its chemical symbol, Hg, is derived from the Greek word *hydrargyrias*, meaning "water silver." At room temperature, the liquid metal releases vapor as a poisonous, odorless, and colorless gas. The amount that's released increases with the temperature.

Once inhaled, mercury vapor readily passes from the lungs and immediately enters the bloodstream. What's not stored in the blood cells quickly diffuses into other cells and tissues throughout the body. Mercury can poison and kill virtually every cell. No matter where in the body it is located, this particular heavy metal is harmful for as long as it is present.[1]

You probably recall the Mad Hatter character in the book—and numerous movies—*Alice In Wonderland*. As a child I knew that the Mad Hatter was one crazy dude, but I didn't learn until I was a bit older the true origins of his name. In the nineteenth century, mercury was used in the manufacturing of hats. After years of breathing in this dangerous heavy metal, hat makers—or hatters—would often suffer from serious nervous system disorders that would cause them to tremble and appear insane.

Toxic Metals and DNA Repair

The most dreadful curse to befall living cells is to be exposed to heavy metals such as lead, cadmium, or mercury. The damage, incapacitation, and impossibility of cell repair are unpleasant even to contemplate.

These toxic metals mount a multifaceted attack, destroying biological entities and systems throughout the cell, and mercury is the worst because it is the most devastating. The first strike is to induce the full gamut of reactive oxygen species (ROS)—hydroxyl radicals, superoxide radicals, and hydrogen peroxide, along with nitric oxide—to damage and destroy the cell. Next, the antioxidant defenses of the cell are attacked when mercury binds directly to active sulfhydryl sites, incapacitating even glutathione peroxidase, the body's most powerful antioxidant enzyme. Every atom of mercury irreversibly consumes up to two molecules of glutathione, increasing the risk of cell damage and degenerative disease.

These now-unchallenged ROS have the upper hand in rendering virtually all the other cellular components dysfunctional. They also can destroy the integrity of the important cell membranes.

Hence the term "mad as a hatter."

Mercury is only one of the poisonous heavy metals wreaking havoc on our health, yet it happens to be many times more poisonous than arsenic, lead, or cadmium. The tiniest amount of mercury, once absorbed by the body, can inflict widespread damage to cells, tissues, and organs. Mercury has a high affinity for nerve cells and readily enters the brain. Once inside the brain, it has a particularly destructive effect on the nerve cells.

Fortunately, some symptoms related to mercury toxicity will diminish or disappear completely when mercury sources are removed. Improvement is even greater when source removal is combined with a detoxification program designed to pull out the mercury stored in your body.[2]

One dark side of mercury is that it is used in hundreds of products we find on the market today. Consumers just don't know it's there. Mercury is found in antiseptics, batteries, cosmetics, diaper products, electric switches, energy-efficient lights, fabric softeners, floor wax and polish, paints, perfumes, photography supplies, tattooing inks, wood preservatives . . .[3]

The list seems endless.

A Dental Biohazard

Millions of people are being exposed to mercury through their workplaces, the products they use, and their diets. But what seems *truly* mad is that the most toxic, nonradioactive, heavy metal on the planet is placed inside the

---

The final assault of ROS drives the cell either to become cancerous or to die through cellular suicide.

Mercury also inhibits key enzymes in the cell's ATP-producing mitochondria, the source of all the cell's energy. With an insufficiency of ATP energy, any remaining membrane integrity is lost and calcium entering the cell triggers the final events of death for the cell. Under the microscope the process is almost painful to observe: cytoplasmic swelling, chromatin clumping, membrane blebbing, and mitochondrial engorgement are grotesque.

The final stage of cell death is unmistakable, as the cell ruptures and its contents are spilled into the intercellular space.

mouth as part of a medical procedure. In fact, the most common source of exposure to mercury is dental fillings.

When I was a boy, I played with a ball of mercury I took from a thermometer that had broken in my dad's lab. We knew back then that it was toxic, so we used a sheet of paper to pick up the liquid metal ball and roll it around and around. Dentists know that the same thing is true when handling the material they use to make fillings, treating the dangerous material as the biohazard it really is.

{
If you have a mouth full of mercury fillings, you create enough mercury vapors—every time you chew—that the environment in your mouth exceeds OSHA standards.
}

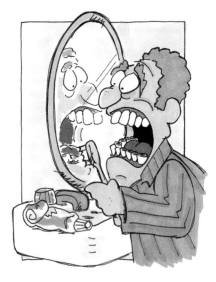

Yet they still put it in your mouth.

It's a lie to say that the mercury becomes stable when placed as a filling. If you have a mouth full of mercury fillings, you create enough mercury vapors—every time you chew—that the environment in your mouth exceeds Occupational Safety and Health Administration (OSHA) standards. You wouldn't be allowed to work in a room that contained that much mercury vapor. And yet we release these vapors and absorb them sublingually—entering the blood through the tissues in the mouth—or breathe them into our lungs, where they travel to our brain.

The American Dental Association (ADA) has issued warnings about removing fillings because the heat of the dentist's drill releases mercury vapor and pieces of mercury fillings may be swallowed. If heating mercury fillings is an issue, we should also be concerned about those fillings being heated by the friction of chewing or while drinking a hot cup of coffee or tea. And because the life of a mercury filling is approximately seven to fifteen years, eventually most fillings fall out and can easily be swallowed.

Your dentist treats removed fillings similar to handling nuclear waste. Then what is this material doing in your mouth?

The FDA Admits Mercury Fillings Pose a Serious Risk

After years of negotiations and stalling, the U.S. Food and Drug Administration (FDA) finally admitted in 2009 that mercury from amalgam dental fillings may be toxic to children and developing fetuses. The admission came when the FDA settled a lawsuit filed by Moms Against Mercury and others concerned about mercury exposure. As part of the court settlement, the FDA agreed to alert consumers about the potential health risks on their Web site.[4]

Mercury Safety Paradox	
Organization	Opinion
FDA	☠
OSHA	☠
ADA (For Dentists)	☠
ADA (For You)	☺
WHO	☠

This court ruling is a necessary first step in completely banning the use of mercury for all medical and dental procedures. But the use of mercury amalgams in dental fillings continues, despite a steady decline due to public awareness.

Mercury is a poison, and it has no place in the mouths of humans. Yet the ADA has historically denied that any harm is being done through the use of mercury in dental fillings, despite a wealth of evidence to the contrary. But when you think about it, how could they admit mercury fillings cause Alzheimer's, Parkinson's, and many other diseases? If they admit this, they would lose all credibility and the lawsuits would be never ending.

From their point of view, they are better off continuing the lie until all mercury amalgams are slowly phased out.

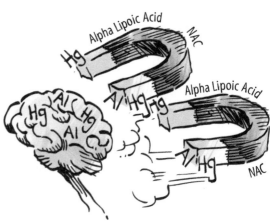

Heavy metals are of serious
concern not only because of
their devastating effects on
the body but also because of
their *persistence* in the body. If
you block all sources of current
exposure to heavy metals like
mercury but do nothing to support
your body's ability to remove it, the accumulation will take years—perhaps a
lifetime—to be eliminated.

The fact is that mercury is removed atom-by-atom through the actions
of the body's natural detoxification systems, including several powerful
antioxidants—substances manufactured by our cells or supplied through
our diet—that reduce oxidative damage. Some antioxidants can chelate, or
bind, with the poison to remove it from the cells and carry it out of the body.
However, if you are deficient in antioxidants, if the detoxification systems of
your cells are impaired, or if there is simply too much mercury entering your
body, this elimination process can be overwhelmed and shut down.

Fortunately, if the sources of contamination are removed and our
bodies' detox systems are given optimal nutritional support, the detoxification
can be accelerated.

Simple Solution:
If you've been exposed to mercury,
consider taking a supplement
containing N-acetyl-L-cysteine
(NAC) and alpha lipoic acid to aid
in detoxification.

If this information is new to you,
then hopefully it's increased your concern
about the dangers of mercury and how
your amalgam fillings affect your health
and the health of those in your family
who have them.

Anyone who knows Dr. Wentz even casually is aware that he is
passionate about banishing mercury amalgams from dental fillings. He

researched and wrote the book *A Mouth Full of Poison* in 2004 to raise awareness of this dangerous medical practice and its impact on our health.

When he learned just how dangerous mercury fillings really were, everyone in our family had our silver fillings removed and replaced with safer biocompatible alternatives. Next, we followed a mercury-detox program with the support of nutritional supplements that would help to rid the body of the mercury that had accumulated.

Whether you have a mouth full of silver fillings or a single glint at the very back, you can reduce your exposure as well. Work with a biological dentist to get all your mercury amalgams safely removed and replaced with biocompatible fillings. If money or time is an issue, ask your dentist to keep a close watch on your mercury fillings and safely replace them—one at a time—as they get older.

{
Work with a biological dentist to get all your mercury amalgams safely removed and replaced with biocompatible fillings.
}

You can also reduce your exposure to mercury at the dinner table. Although you may love sushi, you'll want to stop eating the most mercury-contaminated fish species, such as tuna and swordfish. Instead, get your essential fatty acids from a purified omega-3 supplement like fish or flaxseed oils.

To learn more about mercury go to www.myhealthyhome.com/mercury. To assess your mercury exposure, read Dr. Wentz's book *A Mouth Full of Poison.*

Chapter 6
Don't Be a Dope

Every morning, regardless of what awaits our full attention in the coming hours, we must think of ourselves as our body's CEO.

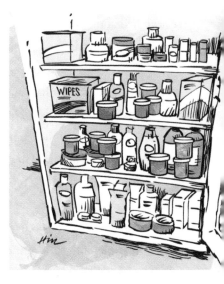

We are faced with daily decisions that have long-lasting ramifications. How should we treat or prevent our ailments? With antibiotics, vaccinations, antibacterials, prescription drugs, and over-the-counter pain relievers and antacids? Or with a little common sense and our own immune system?

As any good business strategist, we must look beyond the temporary, easy fixes and make sound investments in our health—ones that will offer lasting rewards in the long run.

QUIZ

How Toxic Is Your Home?   Scores

1. Which of the following products do you regularly use that contain triclosan or other antibacterial ingredients? (Select all that apply)

   ☐ Hand sanitizer (6 pts)   ☐ Antibacterial spray (6 pts)
   ☐ Antibacterial soap (3 pts)   ☐ Antibacterial toothbrush (3 pts)
   ☐ Antibacterial wipes (4 pts)

2. Do you get a yearly flu shot? Yes_____ (8 pts)

3. How many old, unused prescription drugs are you saving in your medicine cabinet for a rainy day? (5 pts each)

4. When do you reach for pain medicine like aspirin, acetaminophen, or ibuprofen? (Select one)

   ☐ In anticipation of pain (12 pts)   ☐ If the pain is distracting (2 pts)
   ☐ At the first sign of discomfort (8 pts)   ☐ If the pain is unbearable (0 pts)

5. How many over-the-counter or prescription drugs (cough syrup, antihistamines, nasal sprays, etc.) do you usually take when you get a cold? (3 pts each)

Your "Dope" danger score [   ]

1–15	16–30	31–45	46+
Drug-free	Recreational user	Gateway to overuse	Addict

Fighting Germs

With the discovery and widespread use of antibiotics and vaccinations in the past century, we've quickly become a society that seeks to combat every bug that comes our way. Although medical advancements and much higher standards for hygiene have helped us make great strides against serious infectious diseases, we must consider the trade-offs of our unnatural war against germs, a war my microbiologist father will tell you we cannot hope to win by trying to sterilize the planet.

Antibiotics

Most of us catch a cold three or four times a year, and the children in our lives get sick even more often. The symptoms vary—stuffiness, a scratchy or sore throat, earaches, coughing, sneezing, running noses. What never changes is that we feel miserable and want to recover *immediately*.

A huge number of people find the idea of hunkering down for a week or more while dealing with inconvenient viral symptoms unacceptable. So they go to the doctor's office, where they sniffle their way into a prescription for antibiotics. Or they open their medicine cabinet where an old, half-used bottle of Amoxicillin awaits.

"Finally," the cold sufferers think, "I'm going to feel better." A few days later, when the cold virus has run its natural course, they really do feel better, thus reinforcing their mistaken belief that antibiotics are a wondrous cure-all. It's a sad but simple truth that the antibiotics did nothing to help and very likely put the antibiotic abusers—and the rest of us—at risk.

Building the Frankenstein Bacteria

Antibiotics fight *bacterial* infections and do nothing to help cure *viral* infections, such as the common cold, flu, and most upper respiratory illnesses. Many of us prefer to "play it safe," taking an antibiotic "just in case" it will help. In doing so, we've become unwitting collaborators in creating antibiotic-resistant bacteria.

A bacterium can be a remarkably adaptive creature when it comes to surviving in nature—and in our bodies. Bacteria—like most living things—naturally include variants that allow them to survive under changing environmental conditions. When a person takes an antibiotic, the drug kills most of the defenseless bacteria but can leave behind a small number of microbes that have a natural resistance to the drug. These renegade bacteria then rapidly multiply, increasing their numbers a thousandfold in a day and then becoming the predominant microorganism.

Due largely to the irresponsible use of antibiotics, almost every major type of bacterial infection has become less responsive to antibiotic treatment when it's really needed. You've probably heard on the news about forms of tuberculosis and staph infections that are now resistant to drugs, making these diseases much more dangerous and more expensive to treat. These bacteria can quickly spread among hospital and nursing home patients as well as healthy family members and coworkers.

Though the formation of resistant bacteria is a natural process, we can slow it down by reducing our antibiotic use. That means taking antibiotics *only* when they are truly necessary. We also need to take antibiotics correctly when they are prescribed. We shouldn't stop taking our drugs a few days early because we're feeling better; it's almost a sure bet that the strongest, most resistant bacteria will then survive and thrive. As a result, we'll very likely get sick again and, this time, require a stronger, more expensive drug.

So take antibiotics *only* when they are prescribed and absolutely needed, and take them *properly*.

Drugs in Our Food

Even if you're someone who doesn't misuse antibiotics, you may be getting a daily dose without even knowing it.

According to a recent special report by the Associated Press, the United States used about thirty-five million pounds of antibiotics in 2008, and 70 percent of those drugs went to the cows, chickens, and pigs we eat every day.[1] Antibiotics aren't just used on sick animals; they also are administered to healthy livestock to help speed growth. Food animals are typically given the same types of drugs that humans take, which means livestock are major contributors to the problem of antibiotic-resistant bacteria.

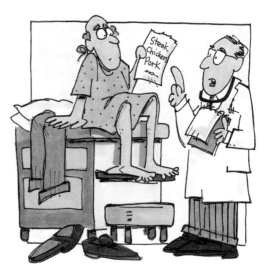

Every time you eat meat, you are most likely drugging yourself with antibiotics.

But wait—antibiotics aren't just sitting on your dinner plate. They're also in your drinking water due to run-off from agricultural operations.

"It's the new prescription for antibiotics."

{ Every time you eat meat you are most likely drugging yourself with antibiotics. }

Powerful agricultural and drug lobbies exert enormous influence on our legislators and government regulators, which means it's up to consumers to protect themselves. You can start by purchasing only organic, antibiotic-free, hormone-free meat. It will be more expensive, but it's time to ask yourself what you're *really* getting when you buy that incredibly cheap pork roast or chicken breast in the store.

The term "killer deal" takes on a new meaning.

Simple Solution:
Give your immune system a boost with the beneficial bacteria found in a probiotic supplement. Just be sure to look in your pharmacy or grocery store for a product that contains "live and active" cultures.

And if you find that the expense makes you cut down on your meat consumption, well maybe that's not such a bad thing either. Remember, grocery stores and their suppliers will follow the money. You can become a serious advocate for food quality by purchasing only healthy, antibiotic-free meat.

Antibacterial Products

With CNN offering minute-by-minute commentary on the latest flu reports and cleaning agent advertisements showing us the microscopic bacteria lurking everywhere in our homes, it's obvious we've become increasingly paranoid about germs. But you don't have to turn on the TV to figure that out. Look around your airport, school, workplace, public buildings, and stores—triclosan-based antibacterial products are everywhere!

Triclosan is a synthetic antibacterial agent now being included in scores of consumer products such as deodorants, cosmetics, acrylic fabrics, plastics, nearly half of all commercial soaps, and even toothpastes. However, a recent analysis performed at the University of Michigan School of Public Health demonstrated that using soap containing triclosan is no more effective in preventing infectious illness than washing with plain soap.[2]

Questions have also been raised about potential health risks posed by triclosan.

First, the combination of triclosan with chemicals commonly found in tap water, such as chlorine, can form dangerous toxic substances including dioxins and chloroform gas. Triclosan has also been linked with liver and inhalation toxicity, and it may disrupt thyroid function. The Environmental Protection Agency (EPA) considers triclosan a pesticide, and when the chemical was introduced in 1972, its use was restricted to health-care settings, such as in a surgical scrub. Today, however, triclosan is found everywhere in American households and workplaces.

Second, such widespread use of an antibacterial such as triclosan is likely to encourage the resistance that bacteria exhibit to antibiotics. Instead of wiping out bacteria randomly—the way regular soap or alcohol-based products do—triclosan may inhibit the growth of bacteria in a way that leaves behind a larger proportion of resistant bacteria.

Third, antibacterial products can actually inhibit the immune system, especially in young children. Our bodies naturally make antibodies, and they do it in response to exposure to bacteria and viruses. Those antibodies remain in our bodies and prevent us from getting sick again from the same virus.

When infants are kept in nearly sterile environments, they miss out on the chance to build up those valuable antibodies that they'll need later in life to fend off illnesses.

With few proven benefits and many potentially serious health hazards, everyday antibacterial products are losing their luster. You don't need an antimicrobial toothbrush, and your children don't need to play in the sterile equivalent of an operating room.

In fact, it may do them harm.

Vaccines

This topic doesn't necessarily occur in the home, but it relates to the drugs you find in your medicine cabinet. It's just as important to your health and well-being—and *especially* to the health of your children.

Simple Solution:
Avoid buying products that contain triclosan and its chemical cousin, triclocarban. Simply wash your hands with regular soap and water to get rid of germs.

The birth of our first child was cause for celebration for Reneé and me. Yet Andrew's arrival was also the culmination of several months of research and serious soul-searching.

Our long deliberations weren't over the color to paint the nursery or even names for our son. Instead, we wondered and worried about whether or not to vaccinate him. More parents are beginning to ask this controversial question, and many have come to the same conclusion that we did.

No vaccinations.

It's an issue that's fraught with fears on both sides, which is why it's important that parents are informed. With an awareness of the risks and benefits of vaccinations, you can make the decision that's best for your family.

What's in That Shot?

TRUE OR FALSE? An act of Congress has given vaccine manufacturers protection from most liability claims and civil suits for injury or deaths caused by vaccines.

True. (You may be detecting a pattern in these "true or false" questions.)

Most people assume that today's vaccines have been thoroughly tested for safety and efficacy before being administered to the public.

They have not.

Not a single study exists to show that vaccinations are safe over the long term, and no comprehensive studies have been done on the cumulative effects of multiple dosing with vaccines.[3] And now that the U.S. government has ensured their own financial "immunity," manufacturers have little incentive to spend money or time on safety studies.

Though the question of effectiveness for various vaccines remains an issue of debate, the evidence of *harm* from vaccinations is accumulating. There

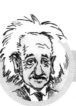

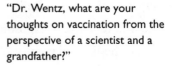
Ask the Scientist

"Dr. Wentz, what are your thoughts on vaccination from the perspective of a scientist and a grandfather?"

I have taken my share of criticism for voicing opposition to recent vaccination campaigns. It is a complex and controversial subject.

The human immune system is incredibly powerful at protecting the body against all kinds of threats, both from the inside and outside. It's logical to think that presenting a foreign antigen to the immune system to stimulate antibody production could enhance this natural power. Unfortunately, strategies employed in implementing this concept have been poorly formulated and irresponsibly administered.

As an immunologist, I have to say that it is a good idea gone wrong.

Instead of taking an antivaccine stance, I like to think of myself as provaccine safety and effectiveness. The words and concepts "vaccine" and "vaccination" do not necessarily have to mean injection. If we hope that a vaccine will effectively bolster the immune system and not interfere or damage it, the vaccine should be administered via a natural route, almost always orally or nasally. Also, adding unsafe toxic materials to a vaccine to make it easier to manufacture and increase its shelf life makes no sense to me.

are many examples of children contracting from a vaccine the very illness it was meant to prevent. There is also overwhelming evidence that certain vaccines can be extremely harmful, causing disability and even death.[4] And vaccines don't necessarily prevent people from getting the disease later in life. Just because you received the measles vaccine doesn't mean you won't get the measles. Vaccines only provide temporary immunity, versus the lifetime immunity developed if the body's immune system fights a disease on its own.

However, the greatest issue I have with this topic is the misguided childhood vaccination program in the United States. To assault the immune system of newborns before the blood-brain barrier has formed (at about two months) and before the immune system has matured (at two years)—resulting in brain inflammation and long-term damage to the immune system—is, in my view, unconscionable.

If you catch a disease and fight it off, the result is far more effective than any vaccine.

The greatest concern when it comes to vaccination is the long-term risk posed by the numerous additives found in vaccines. They contain viruses or bacteria, of course, but they also deliver a dose of detergents and toxic preservatives such as formaldehyde, aluminum, and mercury.

One of the vaccine preservatives you may have heard about is thimerosal, which contains nearly 50 percent ethylmercury by weight. We've already covered in this section the dangers mercury poses to our teeth, so it should come as no surprise that mercury-containing vaccines are extremely dangerous, having been linked to a dramatic increase in neurological disorders, including autism. In fact, autism was first identified as a disorder in children in 1943, just a few years after a mercury-based preservative was added to vaccines.

There's far greater cause for concern about autism than about measles or mumps. Again, a strong immune system is the best defense and cure for these infectious illnesses.

Fifty years ago, autism affected fewer than 1 in 10,000 families. Today, the disease strikes 1 in 100 children.[5] What has changed in fifty years?

Although federal authorities and some studies contend that there is no established link between mercury-based vaccines and autism, the mounting evidence of adverse effects has moved many states to ban the use of thimerosal. Let's not forget, though, that in the case of a "national health crisis," those bans on thimerosal went out the window. In 2009 federal officials gave thimerosal the all-clear in their rush to get swine flu vaccinations to market. It seemed as if they were far more concerned about preventing a public relations nightmare than a flu pandemic.

Though we should applaud forward-thinking government officials for their move to eliminate mercury from most vaccines, we're left with unanswered questions about the new preservative of choice: aluminum.

Is it that much better or just less political?

Unnatural Immunity

Prior to 1989, each U.S. preschooler received eleven vaccinations for polio, diphtheria, pertussis, measles, mumps, and rubella. A decade later, they were receiving twenty-two vaccinations by the time they reached first grade. Today, it's not uncommon for children to receive as many as *fifty doses* of vaccines during their formative years, a time when the developing immune system is most vulnerable.

The fact is that an unvaccinated child would never contract all the diseases for which he or she will be vaccinated. But by being vaccinated— exposed to the diseases contained in the vaccines—a child is forced to mount a coordinated response to multiple diseases, often all on the *same* day. In the case of the Hepatitis B vaccine, infants typically are given their first of three doses on the very day of their birth.

Vaccines also bypass the body's natural defenses and deprive us of the chance to develop a natural immunity to common diseases, a system borne from evolutionary adaptation. Mass vaccinations basically have robbed human development of a valuable natural infection response.[6]

For most parents, the decision of whether or not to vaccinate is a daunting one. We all wonder if our actions will unintentionally cause harm to our child.

> Mass vaccinations basically have robbed human development of a valuable natural infection response.

Unfortunately, the fact that the global pharmaceutical industry has such vast control over the funding and direction of vaccination research means that we may never be able to trust their studies. Until we receive *independent* scientific studies relating to the effects of vaccines over the long term, we're not going to receive credible answers to our nagging questions.

In the meantime, we have a few suggestions that may help, whether you choose to vaccinate or not.

It's Okay to Say "No"

There are certain inalienable rights of which you need to be aware:

- Know that no one has the right to vaccinate you or your child without or against your consent.
- Amend medical treatment forms *before* Mom goes into labor. (Remember, the Hepatitis B vaccination is given on the day of birth.)
- When it comes time to enroll your child in school, seek a legal exemption from vaccination based on philosophical, religious, or medical reasons.

Go to www.myhealthyhome.com/vaccines for information on vaccine waiver forms in the United States and Canada.

Here are some key things you will want to consider:

- If you decide to vaccinate your child, wait as long as possible so his or her immune system has a chance to develop. Two years is recommended.
- Whenever possible, opt for a nasal spray vaccine rather than the injection.
- Do your best to have only one vaccination administered at a time.
- Be certain that the injection is thimerosal-free.

Be a vocal advocate on behalf of your child's long-term health. Again, remember that nobody can make vaccination decisions for you.

The Truth about Cholesterol

No other topic in nutrition or biomedicine suffers from as much misunderstanding and misinformation as cholesterol. So it's important that we do what we can to set the record straight.

Why bring up cholesterol here in the bathroom instead of in the kitchen? Because society's current obsession with cholesterol can be found in millions of medicine cabinets in the form of statin drugs.

What Is Cholesterol?

Before we can talk about the drugs many of us take to control our cholesterol levels, we really should understand just what this much-maligned substance really is.

Cholesterol is a lipidic (or fatty), waxy steroid found in the cell membranes and transported in the blood plasma. Not very exciting, considering all the controversy, but there's far more to cholesterol than what first meets the eye.

The truth is that the body needs cholesterol. This special building block provides a balance of stability and flexibility to all cell membranes. Almost every cell in the body manufactures cholesterol to maintain membrane permeability and fluidity.[7] Without cholesterol, not even mature red blood cells

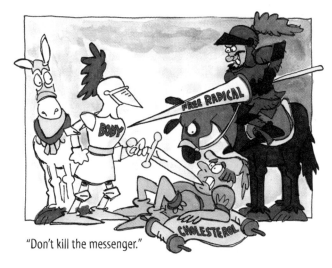

"Don't kill the messenger."

could survive the journey around the body's circulatory system, squeezing through the capillaries as they deliver life-giving oxygen to all the tissues.

Even as cholesterol itself plays such an important structural role in the cell membrane, once it enters any of several biochemical pathways, it gives rise to other compounds essential to life. In the liver, cholesterol is converted into bile salts. Bile salts are stored in the gallbladder until the digestive system needs them. The salts dissolve fats and aid in the absorption of fat molecules in the digestive tract as well as the fat-soluble vitamins: A, D, E, and K.

In the adrenal glands, cholesterol is also a precursor for synthesizing vitamin D and numerous important hormones, including cortisol, aldosterone, and the sex hormones progesterone, estrogens, and testosterone.[8]

No cholesterol, no sex.

Personally, I'm a big fan of cholesterol.

In the skin, cholesterol is secreted by glands just below the surface to protect against dehydration and the wear and tear of sun, wind, and water.[9] Cholesterol is also involved in healing wounds and protecting against infections.[10]

Finally, cholesterol can stand in to perform an antioxidant function when certain vitamins and minerals are in low supply. However, cholesterol is damaged in the process, and oxidized cholesterol *is* bad for the body, whether your cholesterol levels are high or low. That's why getting antioxidants in a steady supply throughout the day is so important. Let your vitamins and minerals protect you from free radicals so they can allow your cholesterol to play all of its other life-saving roles.

What Cholesterol Is Not

Cholesterol is not a poison that will kill you when you consume it as part of your diet.

In fact, even if you eat only food that contains absolutely *no* cholesterol—which is very difficult unless you're a strict vegetarian, as even four saltine crackers or four chocolate chip cookies contain 5 mg of cholesterol, and a serving of rice pudding contains 15 mg[11]—your body will insist on manufacturing at least 1,000 mg of pure cholesterol each day. Why?

Because it needs it—badly. It needs cholesterol to survive.

It's fairly easy to identify foods that don't contain cholesterol. Any food that is unprocessed plant food—fruits, vegetables, whole grains—is cholesterol-free. The reason foods from plants don't contain cholesterol is that cellulose—fiber—is the substance that plants use for cellular structure in place of fats such as cholesterol.

It seems evident that the amounts of any substance naturally synthesized by all the cells individually as well as by organs such as the liver should be carefully controlled by the body. That's why 499 out of every 500 people can control their cholesterol level by nutritional means alone.[12] They don't need pharmaceuticals to do the job.

By itself, cholesterol does not cause cardiovascular disease and stroke. Atherosclerosis is an inflammatory disease. It's what inflammation does to cholesterol that causes arterial plaques. Blaming cholesterol for heart disease is like blaming the forest for the fire that burned your house. Fault the wildfire—or the spark that created it—not the trees. The primary causes of inflammation in general are almost never the presence of too much cholesterol—rather they are too *little* of many other compounds, including essential nutrients, especially antioxidants, B vitamins, and essential fatty acids, as part of a healthy lifestyle.

{ By itself, cholesterol does not cause cardiovascular disease and stroke . . . it's what inflammation does to cholesterol that causes arterial plaques. }

In fact, we probably should be paying more attention to whether our cells and our body contain *enough* cholesterol and ensuring that our cholesterol isn't being damaged by free radicals. That would contribute a great deal to reducing degenerative diseases such as stroke and cardiovascular disease.

Protect Your Cholesterol, Don't Kill It

We've all heard that antioxidants are good for us, but some of us may be a little fuzzy on what they actually do to help us maintain health. Once again, the answer is found in small, chemical reactions on the cellular level that eventually add up to big problems like cancer and heart disease.

Free radicals are the byproducts of chemical reactions in the body—highly reactive compounds that steal electrons from other molecules. (Stick with me here.) Free radical activity can result in a chain reaction that can damage important parts of our cells, such as cell membranes or the DNA in the nucleus. Free radicals are produced during normal body

Simple Solution:
Start with good antioxidant protection, supplemental B vitamins, omega-3 fatty acids, and lots of CoQ10. Also, try one or more of the foods that have been shown to lower cholesterol, such as steel cut oatmeal.

functions, but they also come from exposure to environmental toxins such as air pollution and heavy metals.

When our cells are exposed to unnaturally high amounts of free radical activity, uncontrolled oxidative stress can result. Oxidative stress is associated with virtually every degenerative disease and even the aging process itself. Dietary antioxidants and the antioxidant enzyme systems in our body can quench free radicals and help to prevent the chain reactions that may damage cells.

To continue the forest fire analogy, think of free radicals as a lightning bolt that creates a spark, oxidative stress as the forest fire that can result from that spark, and antioxidants as the park rangers who stamp out the spark before it develops into a wildfire that leaps from tree to tree. It's impossible to completely avoid free radicals, but we can help the body regain balance and reduce oxidative stress by consuming foods such as fruits and vegetables that are high in antioxidant compounds and by supplementing our diet with antioxidant vitamins, minerals, and omega-3 fatty acids.

Statins: Are They Worth the Risk?

One group that surely likes cholesterol is big pharmaceutical companies. In recent years they have made billions of dollars selling statins—drugs that help lower cholesterol levels. These drugs seem to be the latest cure-all for everyone over the age of fifty.

However, even the members of the medical establishment who consider statin drugs the greatest thing since penicillin now acknowledge that these drugs clearly have side effects—as do all drugs—and that the side effects must be taken into account when putting patients on statin therapy.

Hundreds of papers have been published in recent years demonstrating potential health risks, including muscle pain, liver damage, digestive problems, skin rash or flushing, Type 2 diabetes, neurological side effects—doesn't this sound like one of those drug ads? In virtually every case, however, the drugs are given the benefit of the doubt, with the explanation that the benefits of statins far outweigh the risks.[13]

I know one doctor who thinks everyone on the planet should be taking statins, even kids. This stance might be more acceptable if there were no other choice, which seems to be what many doctors assume. They act as if it's a black-and-white matter, with statins on one side, disability or death by heart disease on the other, and a big void in the middle. But this is far from the truth.

Every patient is different, and every case of circulatory disease involves a multitude of factors, from diet to activity level to lifestyle, as well as the genetic diversity of the human race.

Don't forget that cholesterol is an essential nutrient. Driving your cholesterol levels down too far can cause serious health problems. If you have borderline or higher cholesterol levels, you also need to consider other risk factors such as family history of cardiovascular disease, sedentary lifestyle, high blood pressure, age, diabetes, obesity, and your general state of health. However, if you are convinced you should lower your cholesterol levels, there are things that you can do instead of beginning a regimen of statin drugs.

Remember, avoiding heart disease begins and ends with following a healthy lifestyle, *not* with pharmaceuticals. Poisoning your cells' ability to make cholesterol isn't the best way to avoid heart disease.

Cholesterol Lifestyle Solutions

If you want to lower your cholesterol levels, you can make some lifestyle changes that will provide you with other health benefits as well. These include:

- Increasing your fiber intake
- Losing excess pounds
- Getting physical exercise—every day
- Quitting smoking
- Using moderation in alcohol consumption[14]

Self-Medication Nation

As kids, we were constantly told to learn from our mistakes. A cause—attempting to jump a curb on a skateboard—leads to an effect—a bloody nose and nasty road burn. But for some reason, as adults we tend to ignore the relationship between cause and effect when it comes to health problems, preferring to skip personal responsibility and look for easy remedies.

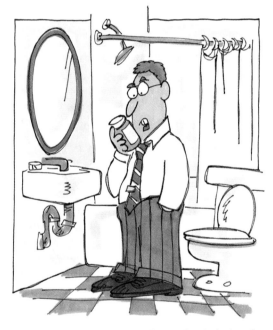

"If I take pain killers now, I won't get a headache later."

Nowhere is this more evident than in our own medicine cabinets.

Today, we medicate every little ache, sniffle, and cough with little

"Dr. Wentz, do I need to be concerned about the effects of drugs on my liver?"

Yes. Because it is our first line of defense in detoxifying poisons, the liver is often vulnerable to sustaining serious damage.

All toxic substances, from pesticides to heavy metals, are directed to the liver from your gastrointestinal tract, your lungs—even your skin—for detoxification. Many of the toxins with which the liver deals become even more toxic after initial processing, but it's still the liver that has to deal with them. The liver may have difficulty metabolizing synthetic drugs—such as some antibiotics—and the unmetabolized compounds can accumulate in the liver, reducing its efficiency. Your susceptibility to liver injury from drugs can be influenced by race, sex, age, and genetic factors.

At one time, alcohol was the leading cause of acute liver disease, but today the single most common cause of drug-induced liver disease is acetaminophen, such as Tylenol®, which is found in more than 700 over-the-counter cough, cold, allergy, and sinus medicines.[15] There are almost 100,000 incidents of acetaminophen poisoning every year.[16]

thought of the long-term consequences to our health. Got a headache? Pop a couple ibuprofen or acetaminophen. Sure, we're probably dehydrated and coming down from our second cup of coffee, but why deal with the cause of the headache when we can just take a pill—or two or three—to numb our senses and hide the painful message our body is sending? Our drug-happy society fails to recognize that the glass of water we're drinking to wash down the pills is likely doing as much to alleviate our headache as the drugs themselves.

Drugs that allow us to do things we really shouldn't—like drinking too much alcohol or eating too close to bedtime—

The seriousness of this problem means that we need to take personal responsibility to reduce drug-induced liver damage. Any drug you take adds to your toxic burden, and taking more than one—mixing medications—exacerbates liver load and damage from interaction products. Alcohol, which the liver must also detox, should *never* be mixed with pharmaceutical drugs.

Be aware of the hazards of the drugs you may be taking and the environmental toxins to which you are exposed. Take care of your liver—so it can take care of you.

without feeling the effects of our actions are a recipe for long-term damage to our health. We need to listen to the body and learn from it.

- We have heartburn because we ate too much. So don't just pop an antacid—*eat less.*
- Our knees ache from over-exertion. So don't take a pain pill in order to continue running—*give them time to heal.*
- We're constipated because we aren't eating enough fiber or drinking enough water. So don't take a laxative and continue bad habits—*improve your diet.*

Remember, we're the ones who pay the price for ignoring our body's signals.

We are seeing reports on many drug-induced diseases—not to mention the crazy, devastating reality of deaths caused by adverse drug reactions. We tune out the lengthy, often horrifying recitation of drug warnings during the commercials or in the full page of miniscule print on the backside of new drug ads in magazines.

But it's time to dial in.

The fact is that when the FDA approves a medication for use by the general public, less than half of the serious drug reactions are known. To find out about the other half, the FDA relies on consumer experiences. Whether we realize it or not, we are the guinea pigs for determining the safety of some of the world's most dangerous drugs.

"If you have purchased recently released drugs or have taken free samples provided by your doctor, you too, are part of this ongoing clinical trial," writes Ray Strand, M.D., in his book *Death by Prescription*. "The use of prescription medication is the third leading cause of death in the U.S. That means an adverse drug reaction is five times more likely to kill you than an automobile accident."

Over half of these deaths can be avoided.[17]

> Whether we realize it or not, we are the guinea pigs for determining the safety of some of the world's most dangerous drugs.

We are vulnerable to the choices made for us by institutions and governmental agencies, but we have more influence than we realize. We can make safe and effective choices when taking prescription medicines or over-the-counter drugs by communicating openly with our physicians about the drugs we are already taking and the new drugs they are prescribing.

Finally, keep in mind what Dr. Strand says about prescriptions: Drugs are a lot like taxes—they are easy to add, but it takes an "act of Congress" to reduce or eliminate them.[18]

The decisions you make regarding your prescription drugs should be made in consultation with your doctor. But you can decide today to cut in half your self-medication with over-the-counter drugs. Before you pop another pill, ask yourself if your headache, stuffy nose, insomnia, or heartburn is really that bad and if you can avoid the symptoms in the future by making simple lifestyle changes.

For more detailed information about medications, visit www.myhealthyhome.com/meds.

That whole cause-and-effect scenario we learned as kids is just as relevant today.

Simple Solutions Summary

The cumulative effect of bathroom toxins demands our heightened awareness. We've touched on just a few of the problems lurking in most bathroom cabinets and drawers, but we hope you've noticed a pattern: Wherever possible, reduce your exposure to toxic products.

Read labels and learn what they mean. Take responsibility for what you put on and into your body, because nobody else will. And most important, don't become discouraged. Making small, incremental changes over time can make a major difference over a lifetime.

What Simple Solutions will you add to your Bathroom?

Scores

1 I will: (Select all that apply)

☐ Find alternatives to products with parabens, formaldehyde-releasers, and other harsh chemical preservatives, especially those that stay on the skin all day (2 pts for every product you discontinue)

☐ Cut the number of personal-care products used each day by 20 percent (8 pts)

☐ Wash products off my face right when I get home in the evening instead of waiting until I go to bed (4 pts)

☐ Cut back on highly scented personal-care products (2 pts for every product you replace with a lightly scented or unscented version)

2 I will: (Select one)

☐ Stop using antiperspirant altogether and replace with natural deodorant (10 pts)

☐ Wash off antiperspirant after I get home (5 pts)

☐ Stop using antiperspirant on weekends and during cooler months (5 pts)

3 I will: (Select all that apply)

☐ Switch to a fluoride-free toothpaste (5 pts)

☐ Begin taking calcium, magnesium, and vitamin D supplements (4 pts)

☐ Switch from mouthwash to a tongue scraper (4 pts)

☐ Rinse with water flavored with a few drops of cinnamon, peppermint, or anise extract instead of mouthwash (3 pts)

4 I will: (Select all that apply)

☐ Safely dispose of all old prescriptions (5 pts)

☐ Commit to listening to the doctor if he or she says I don't need an antibiotic (2 pts)

☐ Reduce antibiotic ingestion by purchasing only organic meats/dairy (7 pts)

☐ Discontinue use of triclosan antibacterial soaps in the home and workplace (6 pts)

5 I will: (Select all that apply)

☐ Talk to the doctor about alternatives to statin drugs, such as lifestyle changes (7 pts)

☐ Begin taking an omega-3 fatty acid supplement (3 pts)

☐ Take a CoQ10 supplement every day (3 pts)

☐ Add a good source of fiber to my daily breakfast (3 pts)

6. I will: (Select all that apply)

☐ Create a list of all the medications and supplements I take to place in my wallet or purse (2 pts)

☐ Take stock of all of the over-the-counter medications taken over the course of the week; look for correlations with lifestyle choices (2 pts)

☐ Eliminate the regular use of at least one over-the-counter medication through behavioral changes—for example, drinking plenty of water to avoid headaches (5 pts for each)

Your Simple Solutions positive score: ☐

Your "Personal" danger score: | - |

Your "Pearly" danger score: | - |

Your "Dope" danger score: | - |

Your Bathroom Health total: ☐

Are you making a positive difference?

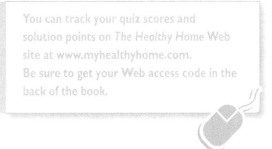

You can track your quiz scores and solution points on *The Healthy Home* Web site at www.myhealthyhome.com.
Be sure to get your Web access code in the back of the book.

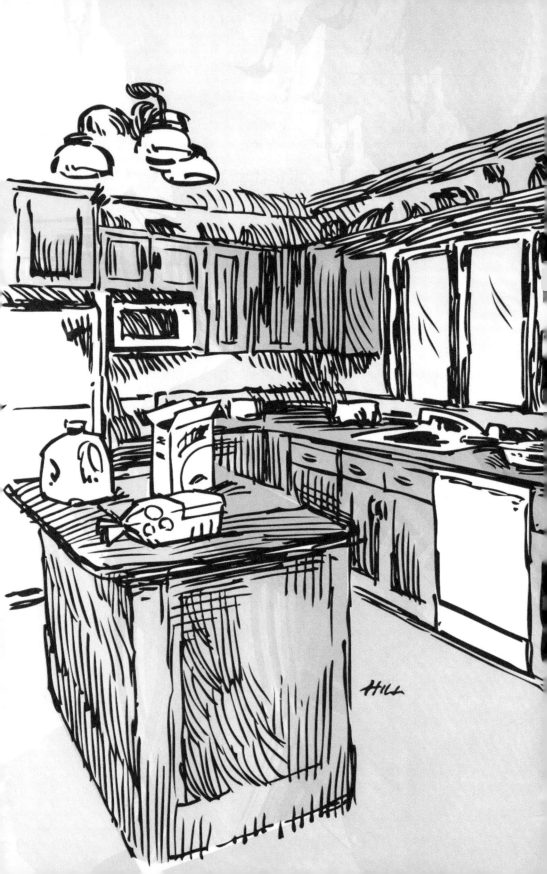

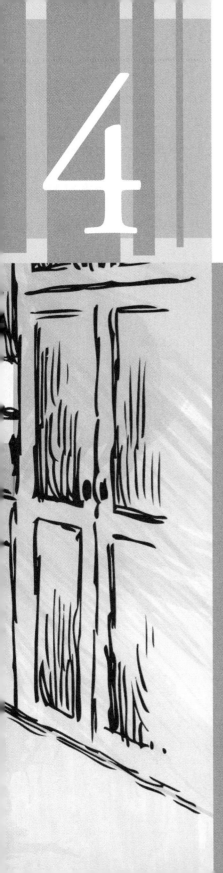

4

The Kitchen

The kitchen is where we come to eat together and share stories of the day. What often proves to be the most chaotic room of the house is nevertheless the hub of our celebrations and cultural traditions, and a place of renewal and restoration for our bodies, souls, and relationships.

Pick up any book on healthy eating and you'll find lots of solid wisdom. But healthy eating encompasses more than what merely goes into our mouths. Simple truths about meals, food preparation and storage, and beverages may be the key to the greatest long-term impact to a family's health.

Simple solutions have never been more readily available . . . or delicious.

Dr. Wentz has a deep passion for healthy eating. Most of his acquaintances would rather have him look in their medicine cabinets or under the bathroom sink than dine with him. The pressure for making the right food choice is enormous. Big, hearty men accustomed to steak and potatoes switch to a salad under his watchful eye.

So it's with some apprehension that we leave the bathroom and head to Dave's kitchen. A brightly lit setting that boasts of gleaming white stone countertops, the kitchen has plenty of workspace and appliances. Yet as with the other rooms we've visited, we can assume that surprising dangers lurk behind those light maple cabinet doors.

Dave: This is actually Reneé's domain. During the renovation, I got my pick of the audio/visual equipment, and she had full control of the kitchen. If I had known how much an oven could cost, though, I might have made a different deal.

Donna: If you're going to do it, I guess you might as well do it right. And it looks as if she did it right.

Dr. Wentz: Yes, this kitchen is impressive, but even so, we cannot underestimate the dangers this room can pose.

Donna: Judging from what we've found elsewhere in the house, it's a safe guess that you're not just referring to touching a hot stove or cutting yourself with a knife.

Dr. Wentz: No, we usually make those mistakes only once or twice in a lifetime. The things I'm referring to are decisions we make every time we sit down for a meal. *[Looking into a cabinet stocked with small kitchen appliances.]* Dave, how *many* gadgets do you have in this kitchen?

Dave: Too many, but some of them were wedding gifts, so you can't really blame me for those. We don't have a deep fryer, and look here—we have a steamer.

Dr. Wentz: With the exception of the steamer, you should be using them all sparingly, and not pulverizing the goodness out of your food. *[Opens a large drawer.]* Glass storage containers—very good. Where's Andrew's drawer?

Dave: Over to your left—you'll find glass baby bottles and bowls, too. I just have to hope they're strong enough to take the punishment, or that I have quick enough reflexes when he starts throwing things.

[Dr. Wentz looks in the trash can and pulls out an object.]

Dr. Wentz: An In-N-Out® bag? Isn't that a fast-food burger place?

Dave: It's something I indulge in every once in a while. We have to allow ourselves the occasional guilty pleasures or else the job of healthy living will become too overwhelming. A fast-food meal is one of the rewards I give myself, but rarely.

Dr. Wentz: Well, at least your pantry isn't packed with a two-year supply of food.

Donna: Do you worry that the food will go bad?

Dave: Not at all. Having *that* sort of supply would mean we were eating a lot of preserved food that had to be processed. The act of doing so would have depleted it of nutrients in order to give it a long shelf life. Dad *prefers* food that goes bad because it's more likely to be unprocessed and healthy.

Dr. Wentz: *[Looking under the sink.]* Dave has a reverse osmosis faucet for the sink, which may be the most critical feature in any home. I've always told him to drink lots of purified water all day—except not with meals.

Donna: But we've all been told, time and again, that we should drink as much water as we can. Why wouldn't we do so at meals?

Dr. Wentz: The problem is that fluids neutralize or dilute the acidic environment of the stomach, which is critical for food digestion and nutrient absorption.

Donna: That's not something people would likely have suspected as a problem. Complexities like that are going to seem daunting.

Dave: I promise it will be less daunting than your average fad diet. We'll focus on some lesser-known issues with the food we eat every day. And we'll show you how everyone can make easy changes that will do the most good.

Chapter 7
For the Love of Food

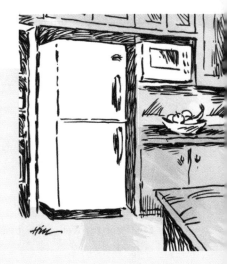

Food is plentiful—at least in most developed
nations. And for the most part, it's cheap and
easy to acquire. Yet we often are left feeling
unsatisfied and wanting more. As a society,
we've developed some serious misconceptions
about what it means to
"dine well."

    Why do we eat?

    We like to party—to eat for fun and
celebration. Some of us eat when we're bored or stressed out. We might even
admit to having a secret addiction to certain kinds of food or drink. And then
there's the real reason to eat—because we need to nourish our body.

QUIZ

How Toxic Is Your Home?   Scores

1. How many brightly colored (red, green, blue, purple, orange, etc.) fruits and
vegetables were on your plate at dinner last night?

3 or more	2	1	0
0 pts	I pt	3 pts	7 pts

2. Which is most similar to what you eat for your typical breakfast? (Select one)

☐ Veggie omelet (0 pts)	☐ Eggs, bacon, and hashbrowns (4 pts)
☐ Whole wheat toast and fresh fruit (0 pts)	☐ Pastry and coffee (7 pts)
☐ Steel-cut oatmeal and fresh fruit (0 pts)	☐ Bagel and cream cheese (6 pts)
☐ Yogurt (4 pts)	☐ Drive-through meal (8 pts)
☐ Candy bar/energy bar (4 pts)	☐ What's breakfast? (10 pts)
☐ Cold cereal (6 pts)	☐ Coffee (15 pts)

3. What do you estimate is the ratio of fruits/veggies to meats/dairy in your diet?

Ratio	10:0	8:2	6:4	5:5	4:6	6:4	8:2	0:10	
Fruits/Veggies									Meats/Dairy
	0 pts	0 pts	I pt	3 pts	5 pts	8 pts	10 pts	15 pts	

4. How often do you go grocery shopping? (Select one)

☐ Monthly (15 pts)	☐ Every 2 weeks (8 pts)
☐ Weekly (I pt)	☐ Every few days (0 pts)

Your "Food" danger score ☐

1–12	13–24	25–36	37+
Gourmet	Fine diner	Fast food junkie	Starving

Modern Dietary Pitfalls

Our society is filled with numerous dietary problems that are evident when we study them at waist level. But what we have chosen to present in this chapter zeroes in on the kitchen and the things we keep there, and it allows us the additional luxury of learning from dinnertime conversations with my family and friends.

We've been duped by food manufacturers and advertisers.

Many of the items we stock in our refrigerators and pantries—the things we've been led to believe will nourish our bodies—aren't really even food. Just because something edible passes our lips doesn't necessarily qualify it as nourishment. Few ingredients in these highly processed poser foods are close to recognizable, and most of the additives—such as coloring, flavorings, and artificial sweeteners—are ultimately toxic. Junk food is deficient and devoid of nutritional value; it's just empty calories that will leave you overfed and undernourished.

And because your body needs the right nutrients to survive, it will keep signaling you to eat. You will experience increased cravings, prompting you to eat more and more.

Dr. Ray Strand, physician and author, has also tackled the topic of food cravings in his book *Healthy for Life*. He describes a food scenario many have personally experienced:

> Think back to a large party or picnic you've recently attended. At one end of the table, the hostess sets a moderately sized bowl of apples, bananas, and oranges (no more than two or three of each). On the other end of the table—in bowls the size of kiddie pools—she pours mounds of chips. She can hardly force those few pieces of fruit on her guests, but she'll definitely have to refill the chips.[1]

We've come to expect it. It's fun to munch chips. The salty crunch factor offers just the right experience.

"Have you ever tried to eat five bananas in a row?" Dr. Strand asks. "I love them, but I can only get one down. On the other hand, have you tried to eat just one potato chip?"

This situation illustrates the difference between what happens when you eat real food compared to junk food. Good foods satisfy. High-quality foods that are nutritionally dense make us feel full so we don't feel the need to overeat. All the others keep us coming back for more. Food manufacturers know it—they count on it. Huge warehouse-sized box stores are a testament to it.

We naïvely fail to question the rapid spread of giant food stores or their far-reaching effects. We see people pushing carts the size of small cars down rows and rows of processed foods. It's little wonder we have to go to the grocery store only once a month.

We have a growing disconnect when it comes to providing nutrition for our bodies. And if it isn't nutrition we're accomplishing, then what is it? We may need to rethink both quantity *and* quality of food.

Marketing Genius

A healthy dose of skepticism will serve us well when shopping for food. We'll find a number of claims that sell the "health-promoting" aspects of a given product, even if the claims are unsubstantiated or if the product inflicts just as many negative effects on our bodies.

For instance, marketers love phrases such as "all natural." But did you know that there's no FDA definition, no legislated standards for using the term? Just about *anything* can claim to be "all natural."

How about "less fat."

Less fat than what? Whale blubber?

Foods can have as much fat in them as the manufacturers want—they just have to have less than at least one other version of the product they are selling. One of my favorite marketing strategies is Diet Coke® putting a giant heart and "The Heart Truth®" on their cans, asking people to support women's heart health programs. Now we can feel good about drinking their chemicals because we're reducing heart disease in women.

Really?

Carbs Are Not Created Equal

TRUE OR FALSE? Eating cold cereal may be bad for your heart.

True.

Popular cereal brands may feature claims on their packaging about how beneficial their products are for heart health. They get away with this because manufacturers focus consumer attention on studies about fiber—which is good for the heart. They then portray themselves as being concerned with health, even though the fiber in their product has been so thoroughly processed that it's rendered useless. More importantly, their product has a number of negatives that they neglect to tell us about.

Advertisers fail to mention that eating highly processed cereal is like pouring table sugar down your throat. This stimulates insulin spikes that over time can contribute to insulin resistance, obesity, and an increased risk of diabetes. Most people know about the damage diabetes can do—damage that may lead to amputation, blindness, and heart trouble. So how have the advertising companies convinced us that eating a bowl of their formulated sugar is healthy?

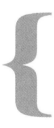

{ Advertisers fail to mention that eating highly processed cereal is like pouring table sugar down your throat. }

This isn't to say that all marketers are liars or all companies are out to sell you harmful products. But it *is* true that you can't always believe what you read. Educate yourself and pay attention to ingredients—not flashy claims.

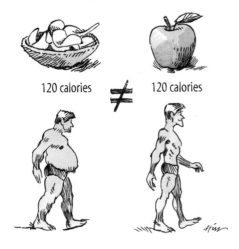

120 calories ≠ 120 calories

Have you ever been short on time and grabbed a donut for breakfast in the morning on your way to work? How did you feel an hour or so later?

Chances are you felt pretty low on energy. What did you crave to eat later in the day?

Most likely, you wanted more sweet carbs. When we eat processed foods—especially flour—the body is being set up. Our bodies absorb these calories very quickly—much too quickly, in fact. The result is a physiological reaction that makes our body crave more. It's similar to having an addiction.

Many of us grew up with the food pyramid. It was probably one of the earliest lessons we learned about nutrition. Now we must *unlearn* what we memorized from cereal boxes, bread sacks, and school lunchroom posters. We should, in fact, *not* be consuming eight to eleven servings of what we then believed were healthy grains, as most of them were bleached and devoid of any nutritional value.

Many of our nation's most popular foods are dangerous because they are highly processed, made with refined flour that comes from high-speed rolling mills that replaced the traditional millstones of the eighteenth century. The new mills became faster and most efficient after the discovery of degermination, a process that took the grain and removed the seed coat—called the bran—and the germ, which is the embryo of the seed that is an integral part of whole-grain foods. It also stripped the flour of a lot of its nutritional value because the bran is where the fiber, B vitamins, and trace minerals are, and the germ contains antioxidants and vitamins B and E.

The impact of this one process forever changed the course of American history, as rarely does an American family go a day without eating bread.

The result of the new milling process was a superfine, pure white flour that does not spoil. How could it get any better for bakers? Not only are the breads and pastries they make from this flour light and tasty, but they also have an extra-long shelf life.

Unfortunately, the results have been less than ideal for those of us who are eating these long-lasting foods. The body is able to absorb the glucose from the superfine particles of white or wheat flour so quickly that it results in a rapid rise of our blood sugar—worse than would occur if you were eating a candy bar. (If only you'd known for all these years that a Snickers® bar would have been better for you than white toast for breakfast!)

And as you know, what goes up must come down. The rapid rise in blood sugar is followed by a rapid fall after a surge of insulin is released to store that sugar in your fat, leaving your fat cells plump and you feeling sluggish. As if that weren't bad enough, you'll also have a seemingly uncontrollable craving for *more* sweets to help get your blood sugar level back in balance.

We are now beginning to realize that our love of pastries and white bread is central to the epidemic of obesity, diabetes, and other inflammatory diseases we see in the world today. Repeatedly eating foods that spike our blood sugar—otherwise known as foods with a high glycemic index—makes us gain weight and, over time, causes lasting damage to our health.

Breaking Bread

Much of the bread you find in supermarkets contains more than flour—much more. Just compare the simple ingredients of good, old-fashioned homemade bread with the ingredients list of the white bread you buy in the store.

Homemade Bread:
Whole-wheat flour, sugar, salt, yeast, milk, butter, and water.

Store-bought White Bread:

Enriched wheat flour, water, wheat gluten, high fructose corn syrup, soybean oil, salt, molasses, yeast, mono and diglycerides, exthoxylated mono and diglycerides, dough conditioners (sodium stearoyl lactylate, calcium iodate, calcium dioxide), datem, calcium sulfate, vinegar, yeast nutrient (ammonium sulfate), extracts of malted barley and corn, dicalcium phosphate, diammonium phosphate, and calcium propionate (to retain freshness).

The Glycemic Index

First introduced by Dr. David J. Jenkins in 1981, the glycemic index has become a household term. Jenkins defined the glycemic index as the rate blood sugar rises after eating a particular test food, relative to that of a control food—usually glucose.

When the glycemic index was first released, most dieticians, nutritionists, and physicians were shocked by the results; it flew in the face of long-held assumptions that complex carbohydrates are always better than simple carbohydrates, and that all calories are created equal.

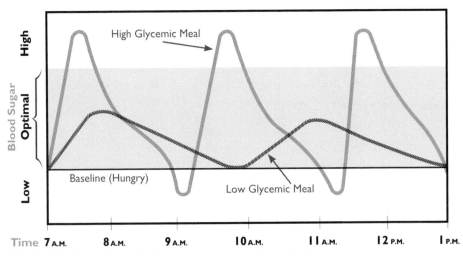

COMPARISON OF GLYCEMIC MEALS

As an example of this new thinking, simple sugars such as table sugar—sucrose—have a glycemic index value of 61, while the sugar found in fruits—fructose—has a much-preferred glycemic index value of only 19. Thus, many of our "healthy" breakfast cereals, such as corn flakes, bran flakes, and oat rings top out the glycemic index, some scoring as high as 92. Suddenly those plastic baggies full of Cheerios® for kids don't seem like such a great snack, unless you want your kids to be chubby enough to stay warm in the winter.

To get an even truer view of your response to a particular food, you'd need to calculate the glycemic load. Glycemic load takes into account the glycemic index *and* the concentration of carbohydrates. Low is 10 or less, medium is 11–19, and 20 or greater is considered high. For example, cooked carrots have a medium glycemic index of 49, whereas their glycemic load is a very low 2.4 because there are few carbohydrates in carrots. This means that eating carrots won't tend to spike your blood sugar. However, potatoes have both a high glycemic index *and* a high glycemic load, which will significantly raise the blood sugar and stimulate a heightened insulin response.

Glycemic Index of Selected Foods

Cereals	GI
Shredded wheat	67
Raisin bran	73
Oat rings	74
Corn flakes	83
Fruit	
Apple	38
Orange	43
Raisins	64
Dates	103
Snacks	
Chocolate bar	49
Potato chips	56
Doughnut	76
Jelly beans	80
Vegetables	
Yam	54
Sweet corn	56
French fries	75
Baked red potato	93
Breads	
Rye	64
Wheat	68
White	70
Bagel, plain	72
Legumes	
Soy beans, boiled	16
Kidney beans, canned	29
Lima beans, boiled	32
Baked beans	45

One of the best ways to avoid high-glycemic carbs is to eat fresh fruits and vegetables deep in color—these are also typically richer in antioxidants. Whole foods that grow close to the ground are packed with living vitamins, minerals, water, fiber, and the enzymes needed to digest the food itself. They are the perfect fit for the cells of our bodies and for nurturing the body in just the right balance.

Find out more about the glycemic index and the glycemic load of specific foods at www.myhealthyhome.com/glycemic.

Thousands of studies have proven that fruits and vegetables are excellent sources of important phytochemicals that are beneficial for fighting disease.

Beyond fruits and vegetables, you can gain control of the glycemic load of your diet by reducing your intake of refined sugars and starches, eating fiber-rich foods, and consuming balanced meals containing protein and fat along with carbohydrates.

Simple Solution:
Garden produce in a rainbow of colors will help you maintain a low-glycemic, nutrient-rich diet. The deeper the color, the better.

Out of Balance

All of life is a matter of balance. Not a frozen balance, like a statue—that would mean death—but rather a delicate balance, which allows moderate movement in one direction or the other, bending but not breaking.

The human body needs this kind of dynamic stability, as do all other living things. The process is called homeostasis, in which internal conditions—like body temperature, blood levels of calcium, and blood pressure—are maintained within narrow ranges, despite the extreme changes that may occur outside.

But most of us today, in the name of convenience, are throwing *out of balance* the complex and overlapping mechanisms inside our bodies.

One of the most important homeostatic mechanisms in the body is the acid-alkaline balance, or pH. Our bodies work hard to maintain a blood pH between 7.35 and 7.45—ideally about 7.40, or slightly alkaline. This is the ideal pH for many of our enzyme systems to work well.

The human body settled on this pH range largely because our early diets consisted of a plant-to-animal ratio of close to 1:1, with fish and shellfish comprising much of the animal component.[2] These diets, high in unprocessed plant fiber and fruits, would have been slightly alkaline, which guided our evolutionary development.

But times have changed, and so have our diets. Profound alterations in humankind's cultural and biological environments, brought about around 10,000 years ago through the introduction of agriculture and animal husbandry, were then magnified with the arrival of the industrial revolution. On an evolutionary scale, such shifts occurred too recently and too swiftly for the human body to adapt. In conjunction with this growing discord between our ancient biology and today's prevailing nutritional and cultural patterns, many of the so-called "diseases of civilization" have emerged[3]— consequences of twenty-first-century diets meeting stone-age bodies.

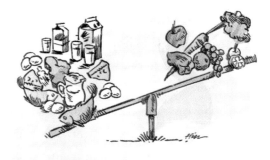

The foods we consume today would have been unrecognizable to our hunter-gatherer ancestors and those first farmers, yet the nutritional needs of our cells have hardly changed at all. Meat products, dairy products, and cereals provide most of the calories in our diets, and they are all high on the scale of acid-producing foods.[4] But remember, our bodies lean toward the alkaline. So we're making it difficult for our systems to maintain the acid/alkaline balance that has prevailed since the beginning of human time.

The basic rule is that meat and dairy foods have a high acid load, whereas vegetables and many fruits are acid-reducing. People frequently confuse the *acidity* of a food source with its *acid load*. It appears paradoxical, but a lemon—which is quite acidic—will actually reduce the body's acid load once its mineral contents—generally found in the pulp—are absorbed into the body fluids. This is because the predominant minerals within the lemon have an alkalizing or acid-reducing effect on the body. They do this by forming mineral hydroxides and carbonates in our cells, which act like molecular sponges to "suck up" excess acidity.

In addition to eating more vegetables, you can also take potassium bicarbonate to help reduce your body's acid burden. But why is it so important to reduce the acid burden of the body and move our diet back to match that of our evolutionary development? Two major risks arise from modern acid-producing diets:

- Osteoporosis
- Cancer

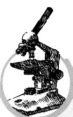

Cellular Truths

Acidity—Your Bones and Cancer

Net *acid load* is an expression that refers to the amount of acid (H^+) the foods we consume contribute to the cells of the body. As such, it represents the total **body burden** of dietary acid. A net acid load of zero would imply that the foods eaten were exactly balanced in their relative acidity and alkalinity. Whereas our ancestral diets were slightly alkaline, today's modern Western diet has a high net acid load.

This has severe implications for long-term bone health.

Through direct chemical dissolution of the bone, bone tissue buffers the acidity of the body. In the process, calcium (Ca^{+2}) and carbonate (CO_3^{-2}) are released from the bone mineral matrix.[5] The release of calcium into the blood and its excretion in the urine are **not** compensated by equivalent calcium uptake from foods in the stomach. Sodium (Na^+), potassium (K^+), and assorted phosphate (PO_4^{-3}) ions also are released from the bone to combine with the excess hydrogen (H^+) in the blood.[6]

Unchecked, this degrading process leads to thinner, weaker bones—osteopenia—and, if not corrected, osteoporosis, or hollowed-out bones.

Acidosis and Bone Health

To protect at all costs the pH balance of the blood, the body sacrifices bone tissue, enlisting the minerals as buffers against the corrosive effects of excess acidity. As little as one week on a mildly acidic diet is sufficient to show a detectable drop in bone minerals from the bone surface.[7]

Consequently, acid-producing diets can dramatically alter both bone structure and function. A high dietary acid load has been shown to both *increase* bone resorption—a process by which the bone structure is depleted—and *decrease* bone formation.[8]

A Cancerous Environment

Everybody has cancer cells. Period. Your mom, your brother, your spouse all have them. Cancerous cells are formed continuously in the human body, with an estimated 10,000 cells active at any given time, but their growth is normally kept in check by an active, healthy immune system.[9] So the question is: Are you feeding these cancerous cells or fueling your body's fight against them?

Recent studies have emerged that provide intriguing insight into the relationship between diet and cancer. Abnormalities in our acid/alkaline balance seem to play a major role in the beginnings of cancer by knee-capping the immune response and allowing cancerous growths to start.[10] High levels of inflammation also block the body's natural defenses by disarming its specialized white blood cells and enhancing the production of chemical-signaling molecules to further inhibit immunity and encourage unchecked

An acid-promoting diet also initiates a broad cascade of biochemical and physiological changes to the body that appear to set us up for cancer. These include:

- Chronic oxidative stress

- Enhanced catabolism— muscle wasting and destruction of skeletal reserves

- Elevation of insulin and cortisol

- Systemic inflammation

- Obesity

- Impaired immunity

Each of these aberrations is known **singularly** to be involved with the genesis of the cancer process. Just imagine the implications when they are **all** pulling on the same rope.

growth.[11] Measuring the level of systemic inflammation can, in fact, predict a patient's survival time for several cancers.[12]

For more science behind acidic/alkaline foods, go to www.myhealthyhome.com/balance.

Respect Your Elders

Although the science of acid/alkaline balance sounds complicated, making your diet more like that of your ancestors is actually quite simple: Consume more whole foods and eat less processed junk.

You can bring pH balance back to the dinner table by serving meals that consist of 60 to 80 percent alkalizing fruits, plants, and vegetables. You'll want to reduce your use of acid-promoting white flour by using whole multigrain flour in its place. You also can increase your intake of inflammation-reducing omega-3 fats, found in fish and flax seeds.

Finally, aerobic exercise every day will help blow out excess acid-producing CO_2 from your tissues and help maintain muscle tone.

Simple Solution:
Start each day with an alkalizing glass of lemon water by squeezing a fresh lemon (no sugar) into purified water. Make sure you include the pulp.

More Potassium, Less Salt (Sodium)

Those pesky ancient ancestors have another message for us in regard to the imbalance of our modern diet: We're getting far too much salt and not nearly enough potassium. It's estimated that our ancestral diet had a potassium/sodium ratio of 10:1, which has now been inverted to 1:3—three times as much salt as potassium—reflecting a thirty-fold change.[13]

Basically, our meals used to feature potassium-rich fruits, vegetables, nuts, and beans along with a small amount of fish or meat—all of which naturally contain only a small amount of sodium.

As bad as sodium can be for us, potassium provides a wide range of benefits that include helping to maintain a healthy blood pressure, rate of metabolism, and muscle strength as well as reducing the threats of anxiety, heart and kidney disorders, and stroke.

Compare that to our modern diet of high-sodium, highly processed food. In that frozen meal or can of condensed soup you had for lunch—maybe with a single serving of veggies—you received up to 1,700 mg of salt. This inverted ratio of potassium to sodium in our contemporary diet is known to adversely affect cardiovascular function and contribute to hypertension and stroke.

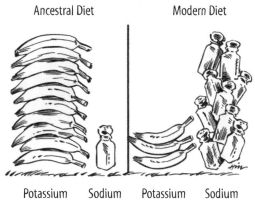

Ancestral Diet   Modern Diet

Potassium   Sodium   Potassium   Sodium

As if that weren't disturbing enough, we've recently learned that high-sodium foods and acid-producing foods can act *independently* to induce and sustain increased tissue acidity. This "tag team" effect is enhanced as you get older and by the kidney's impaired ability to excrete excess acidity.[14]

Even if you never reach for your salt shaker, you could be getting far too much sodium. The best way to decrease your salt intake is to cut back on processed or convenience foods like canned soups, frozen meals, and potato chips. Read your labels. Even if something doesn't *taste* salty, it can contain an entire day's worth of recommended sodium.

Simple Solution:

Trade in your table salt for natural sea salt, which contains a mixture of alkaline complexes. And use pepper or other spices to liven your meals.

Although it's important to reduce sodium levels by cutting back on processed foods and by reducing salt intake, don't forget to increase your potassium, too. Foods rich in potassium include apricots, avocados—break out the guacamole!—bananas, cantaloupe, kiwis, carrots, prune juice, raisins, and more.

Visit www.myhealthyhome.com/potassium for more examples of potassium-rich foods.

Balancing Good and Bad Fats

Earlier we talked about good carbs vs. bad carbs and the need to stay away from those white foods with high-glycemic indexes. Well, we've also gotten seriously out of balance with our fat consumption.

For years, governments and marketers did us a disservice by ranting and raving about getting fat out of our diets. We actually *need* fat—in fact, we can't live without it. Our brain is mostly fat. In our attempts to go "fat-free," though, we mainly reduced the amount of good fat we consume and increased the amounts of sugar and bad fat in our diets.

Some nutrition authorities consider the essential fatty acids (EFAs) the closest

Ask the Scientist

"Dr. Wentz, how did you come to your understanding of the importance of nutrition?"

I believe nutrition is the most important science in all of medicine. My own realization about the importance of nutrition came about as a result of my scientific research. While growing cells for twenty years at my previous company, Gull Laboratories, I learned what nutrients, vitamins, minerals, and cofactors were needed to keep human cells truly robust and healthy.

Later, I learned how much of the nutritional value of our foods has declined over recent decades. We have turned the beautiful world that God gave us into a dumping ground for our toxic wastes, robbing our food of the nutrients we need to stay healthy and exposing our bodies to harmful substances. Because of the environmental hazards in today's society, our bodies—the cells, organs, and systems it comprises— need significantly greater amounts of the essential nutrients, especially the protective antioxidants, than ever before. Nutrition that will help our cells defend themselves from the oxidative stress of today's environment is critical.

There is no question that the nutritional needs of most people's cells simply aren't being met by the food they consume, which is having

thing we have to a true miracle nutrient because they're involved in so many aspects of our health. From cardiovascular disease to autoimmune diseases such as multiple sclerosis and cancer, it would take page after page to note the full listing of the health conditions that we know are influenced by either a deficiency or an imbalance of EFAs.

However, their influences on our health at the cellular level can be grouped into three major categories.

First, EFAs are critical structural components for all cell membranes. The "good" fatty acids—omega 3s and omega 6s—keep the cell membranes flexible, which is important for transporting nutrients and oxygen into the cells and waste products out of the cells.

Second, they are the precursors to important molecules—prostaglandins—that are key to regulating more than a dozen critical functions from inflammation to nerve transmission.

Third, the essential fatty acids are involved in many important processes without which the cells and the body could not survive. For example, fatty acids are needed for oxygen transport from the lungs to the red blood cells that are circulating in the blood vessels. They do this by facilitating the transport of oxygen through the capillary walls, red blood cell walls, and directly to the hemoglobin in the red blood cells.

devastating consequences—a rapidly growing epidemic of chronic degenerative diseases. The good news, however, is that degenerative diseases are diseases of lifestyle, which means they can be prevented through small adjustments in daily habits, such as avoiding environmental toxins and stress, obtaining regular physical exercise, and providing your body with optimal nutrition.

In fact, over the years, I have become convinced that optimal personal nutrition is the single most effective thing we can do to decrease our risk of degenerative disease.

In with the Good, Out with the Bad

To avoid the damaging fats, read your labels.

"Partially hydrogenated" oils of any type are detrimental to your health. These oils contain trans-fatty acids, which most nutrition experts agree are unhealthy for human consumption.

To increase your intake of good fats, look for key phrases on the label:

- Cold-pressed
- Unrefined
- Organic

Use extra virgin olive oil, canola oil, coconut oil, rice bran oil, grape seed oil, or butter for cooking. Eat nuts (almonds/hazelnuts) and seeds (pumpkin/sesame) for snacks. Another good source of healthy fat is flaxseed oil, which can be drizzled over a salad or added to a smoothie.

Food for the Soul

With all of our talk about the importance of good nutrition, let's not lose sight of just how much fun food really is. Yes, food is fuel, but it's also something to be enjoyed and shared.

Take some time every weekend to map out your week's meals. Make planning your menu something fun and encourage the whole family to join in. With a little effort and a little common sense, you can enjoy a healthful diet full of nourishing, clean, real food.

Start wherever you are—nutrition novice or dietary genius—and take it day by day. It's the choices you make consistently every day that will make all of the difference in the long term.

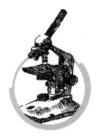

Chapter 8
Let's Get Cooking

The science of food and its ability to sustain life—or steal it—is a fascinating subject and one we never tire of discussing. It's heartening to see how many people have recognized that *what* we eat is incredibly important to our wellness and longevity. But we're also

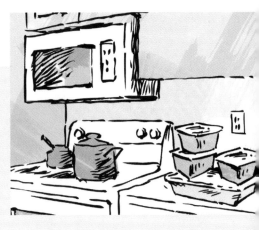

learning that *how* we eat—including how we prepare and store our food—is another significant factor in our nutritional intake and overall health.

QUIZ How Toxic Is Your Home?   Scores

1. Do you use nonstick pans?

Always			Sometimes			Never
10 pts			5 pts			0 pts

2. How do you like your veggies? (Select one)
   - ☐ Raw (0 pts)
   - ☐ Puréed (7 pts)
   - ☐ Cooked but crunchy (1 pt)
   - ☐ Deep fried (10 pts)
   - ☐ Cooked until soft (4 pts)

3. Select the three methods you most often use to prepare your evening meals.
   - ☐ Grill/charbroil (5 pts)
   - ☐ Slow cook (2 pts)
   - ☐ Deep fry (8 pts)
   - ☐ Microwave (1 pt)
   - ☐ Boil (5 pts)
   - ☐ Steam (0 pts)
   - ☐ Bake (2 pts)
   - ☐ Cut raw produce (0 pts)
   - ☐ Sauté/Fry (1 pt)
   - ☐ Call for takeout (8 pts)

4. If you eat steak, how do you typically order or prepare it? If you don't eat steak, enter 0.

Raw (tartare)					Well done
0 pts	1 pt	2 pts	3 pts	4 pts	5 pts

5. What role does plastic play in your kitchen? (Select all that apply).
   - ☐ Plastic or foam containers for heating food in the microwave (8 pts)
   - ☐ Plastic wrap for covering food that's being heated in the microwave (8 pts)
   - ☐ Plastic wrap for covering stored food (4 pts)
   - ☐ Plastic or foam containers for storing food/leftovers (4 pts)
   - ☐ Plastic or foam cups, plates, bowls, etc. (5 pts for each)

Your "Cooking" danger score

1–15	16–30	31–45	46+
Master chef	Line cook	Prep cook	Dishwasher

The Making of a Meal

Let's say you are cooking a nice, homemade meal for your family tonight. First of all, bravo! You've already made a better choice for yourself and your loved ones by not eating out or ordering in. But before you pull out your ingredients and favorite kitchen implements, consider a few things you can change along the way to make that delicious home-cooked meal even healthier.

Due to the widespread nutrient depletion of our topsoil, many of the fruits, vegetables, and grains we purchase today in the grocery store are lower than their predecessors in important vitamins and minerals—and that's before the food reaches your kitchen pantry or refrigerator. Just how much more of

> { The less work you need to do while you're in the kitchen, the more nutrient value your food typically will have . . . reduce the amount of slicing, dicing, cooking, blending, boiling, and peeling. }

the nutritional benefits we lose depends on our culinary methods. The choices you make when storing, cutting, and cooking broccoli, for example, could cut its vitamin C levels by more than half.

One simple rule to remember is that the less work you need to do while you're in the kitchen, the more nutrient value your food typically will have. You also risk creating toxic compounds when food is overcooked or charred. Take it easy and reduce the amount of slicing, dicing, cooking, blending, boiling, and peeling.

A Method to the Madness

Considering the wide variety of food types we're dealing with, there's no single perfect method to follow in the kitchen when it comes to preserving the nutritional content of your food. But some simple modifications to your food preparation methods will minimize nutrient depletion and make you healthier.

Slicing and Dicing

When it comes to slicing and dicing produce, the greater the surface exposure you create, the more key minerals and antioxidants you will lose. For example, slicing carrots in thin, diagonal pieces exposes a larger area of the carrot to the depleting effects of oxygen and to greater leaching through cooking. Think about that sliced apple that browns when exposed to the air even before you can finish eating it.

The section of your grocery store where you find prepared foods will be particularly problematic for this very reason. Although a plastic container of diced melon or sliced carrots *seems* convenient, you're much better off purchasing whole fruits and vegetables and cutting them up just before you eat them.

You'll save money and gain valuable vitamins and minerals.

Simple Solution:
Preserve the nutritional value of your fruits and veggies by cubing them or simply eating them whole. Save the fancy diagonal cuts for cocktail parties.

Steaming

No surprise here: Steaming appears to be one of the best cooking methods for keeping the vitamins and minerals in your veggies, especially broccoli, Brussels sprouts, cauliflower, and cabbage.[1]

Optimize the positive effects by keeping the cooking time to a minimum and ensuring that your vegetables are not immersed in the water. If we steam our food into mush—until it looks like baby food—we lose too many nutrients.

Leave a little crunch in your carrots.

Although steaming is an excellent choice for preparing your food, avoid the "steamer" meals and side dishes found in the freezer aisle of the grocery store. These products are designed to be microwaved in their plastic packaging, which, as we'll learn later in this chapter, carries far greater risks than lost nutrients.

Frying

Though we all know that frying isn't the optimal way to prepare food, this method occupies the middle ground when it comes to preserving antioxidant content.[2] However, this isn't an excuse to make French fries a new food group.

Deep frying—a cooking method most common outside the home—is the biggest no-no there is when it comes to food. Whether it's fries, chicken tenders, or onion rings on the menu, we're likely exposing ourselves to carcinogens and rancid oils. Avoid them like the plague or, at the very least, eat sparingly.

Boiling

Boiling is generally associated with the greatest nutrient losses in meats and vegetables.[3] One study found that the folic acid in broccoli—important for producing healthy red blood cells and reducing anemia—was reduced by 55 percent after boiling. Compare that to steamed broccoli, which has been shown to have no significant reduction in folic acid levels.[4] Nutrient losses from boiling occur mainly when the nutrients are leached into the water,[5] so the addition of a small amount of salt and a reduction of your cooking water can help.[6]

Microwaving

This is an area of great confusion and debate. Some people love it and some hate it. And currently there's just not enough science and information to declare a winner, so we're going to give you both sides of the argument and let you decide.

When food scientists reviewed vitamin and mineral retention in twenty different vegetables, microwaving—like steaming, grilling, and baking—was found to be an ideal method. As with steaming, the less water and time used to microwave the food, the more nutrients were kept. Ensuring an even distribution of heat will also help, and despite what you may have heard, research suggests that microwaves *do not* cause cancer.[7]

The Bad:

The unanswered question is: If electromagnetic fields can alter our cells, will they also alter the energetic integrity of our food? Microwaves are electromagnetic waves, but so far there is very little evidence that they mutate our foods.

Yet the migration of contaminants from the containers that hold the food during heating is of growing concern. Unlike grilling, baking, frying, and steaming, for which you can't use plastic containers because they'll melt, microwaves allow cooking with plastic, and plastic is a known hazard.

In addition, before we fire up a big bowl of our favorite vegetables—or a bag of popcorn, if we're being honest—we should keep in mind that microwave ovens are powerful sources of radiofrequency fields and can leak significant amounts of EMFs. The only way to know for sure *how much* leakage is occurring is to measure the EMFs with

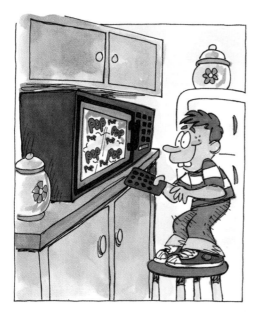

"We are in the final seconds, 4,3,2...it pops, it scores."

an inexpensive Gauss meter, which can be found online or in home improvement stores.

Regardless, if we choose to use a microwave oven to cook, we shouldn't stand and watch it like a television.

Death by Charring

The way you cook your food involves more than just the potential loss of minerals. Some people may like the charbroiled taste, but there's no question that overheating food—no matter what it is—may result in toxic compounds.

Simple Solution:
Maintain a good distance—at least ten feet in front or five feet to the side—between yourself and the microwave when it's on.

In this case, it's not how long you cook your food; rather, it's the temperature you use that can transform healthy nutrients into indigestible chemicals that may threaten your health.

The most obvious example is the all-American backyard barbecue, with steaks, burgers, and hot dogs sizzling on a flaming grill. Cooking meats at high temperatures creates chemicals called heterocyclic amines (HCAs), and exposing meats to direct flames produces polycyclic aromatic hydrocarbons (PAHs), both of which are linked to increased risk of cancer, particularly GI cancers.[8]

Meats are not the only problem. Compounds called acrylamides are present in dangerous amounts in carbohydrate-rich foods that have been overcooked by frying, grilling, or roasting.[9] Found most often in foods such as potato chips and fries, acrylamide is also produced while making toast from some breads.

However, the connection between acrylamides and cancer and other degenerative diseases is less clear than it is for compounds produced by overcooked meats.

, is to keep your cooking temperatures as low as reasonable,

, that are golden rather than brown or black. Even better,

ır diet as many raw foods—such as fruits and vegetables—as you

ι.

ally, monosaturated fats such as canola, flaxseed, olive, and sunflower oils a e better for cooking than polyunsaturated fats, but as soon as you see smoke coming off the oil, you know the temperature is too high.[10] It's not only a fire hazard, but it's also giving your food a bad taste and producing mass of free radicals that will attack your circulatory system.

A Sticky Situation

If you often get dish duty at home, you know the frustration of washing a pot that has remnants of whatever you just cooked cemented to the bottom. You soak and scrub, and scrub and soak. And if you were unfortunate enough to scorch your dinner in that pot, you have an even bigger chore ahead of you.

> { The stuff that lines a nonstick pan and helps your scrambled eggs slide onto the plate is also poisoning your family. }

For that reason, many home cooks have turned to nonstick cookware. After all, you use little to no oil and, like magic, the food comes right off the pan's dark interior. Dish duty suddenly looks a whole lot easier.

But the stuff that lines a nonstick pan and helps your scrambled eggs slide onto the plate is also poisoning your family.

Most nonstick cookware is coated with polytetrafluoroethylene (PTFE), a polymer that a DuPont scientist discovered in 1938 and is considered one of the most slippery materials in the world. PTFE, trademarked by DuPont as Teflon®, can be found today in numerous consumer products, from paint to stain-resistant carpet to electric razors.

At high temperatures, Teflon is known to release potentially hazardous fumes and particles into the air. According to the Environmental Working Group (EWG), a nonstick pan at just 680°F on a regular electric stove released at least six toxic gases, including two carcinogens, two global pollutants, and a chemical that is known to be lethal to humans.[11]

Even at lower temperatures—464°F—the EWG found that toxic particles were released.[12]

These temperatures might sound impossibly high, but the EWG observed that pans can reach 680°F or higher in just a couple of minutes of preheating on a high setting.[13] It's mind-boggling that cookware—with the sole purpose of being placed on a heat source—is lined with something that under high heat emits toxic fumes.

The dangers of nonstick cookware at high temperatures have surprised many unfortunate pet owners who have lost their canaries, macaws, finches, and other pet birds to "Teflon toxicity." Birds that have been poisoned with fumes from overheated PTFE often suffocate after their lungs hemorrhage and fill with fluid.

For this reason, even DuPont recommends that birds be removed from the kitchen before cooking with nonstick pans.[14] (This sounds a little like the toothpaste warning from section 3.) Due to their higher metabolism and more sensitive

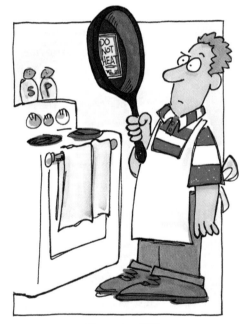

"Do not heat???"

respiratory systems, birds were once used in coal mines as living carbon monoxide detectors. If a canary showed signs of distress, miners knew the air was unsafe and would evacuate.[15]

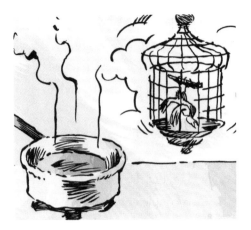

It's time to ask ourselves if we can afford to ignore the metaphorical—and now quite literal—canary in the coal mine . . . or kitchen, in this case.

Healthier Non-Stick Alternatives

Although you may not be able to trash an entire cookware set, you should discard your traditional nonstick pans as they become scratched or dented.

But before you pick up that scouring pad and start scrubbing away again, you should know there are some good alternatives.

First, you can use a well-seasoned cast iron skillet instead. It takes some maintenance but provides great nonstick qualities.

There are also some excellent "green" nonstick pans currently on the market. Many use natural coatings—including ceramic and sand—to create a lasting nonstick surface that contains no PTFE or other harmful chemicals. Several of these new nonstick alternatives have been rated as high as or higher than their

> **Simple Solution:**
> If you must use a PTFE-lined pan, keep your stove's burner on medium or lower. Also, never preheat an empty pan.

PTFE-lined counterparts for durability, nonstick surface quality, and the even the way in which they cook.

For all of you late-night snackers and movie watchers, microwave popcorn bags are also coated on the inside with toxic nonstick chemicals to help the popcorn slide right out. If you can't live without this salty snack, consider purchasing an air popper or old-fashioned popcorn popper.

It's not much more work, and the popcorn tastes better.

Our Plastic Kitchen

Take a look around any room in your home and you'll easily spot dozens of items that contain plastic: carpet fiber, clothing, even the paint on your walls. In less than a century this man-made material has become an indispensable part of our daily lives.

However, it also has the potential to compromise our health.

I've certainly given plastic—and its environmental impact—plenty of thought in the past fifteen years. After all, I run a company that packages most of its products in some form of plastic. The safety and quality of our finished product is our top priority, but we also strive to follow sustainable practices and actively seek viable alternatives to plastic packaging. Yet it was the birth of my son that made my professional interest in plastic become a much more personal concern.

Recent news stories have called attention to Bisphenol A (BPA), a chemical found in certain hard plastic products—including some baby bottles—that are linked to neural and behavioral problems in infants. The idea that I might feed my son with a bottle that could hurt him was disturbing, to say the least. So I set out to learn as much as I could about plastic:

- How it's made
- What types are safest for my family
- Where I could easily reduce our risks in the home

I found that it was in the kitchen—where plastic is used to store, prepare, and serve the food and liquids we consume each day—that I could most easily make a positive impact.

What Is Plastic?

Plastic is a common term for a huge range of synthetic and semisynthetic solids, including nylon, PVC, polystyrene (Styrofoam), and polycarbonate. The most common raw materials used to manufacture plastic are crude oil and natural gas, from which compounds are extracted and eventually linked into flexible chains (polymers). In final processing, plastics often are modified with chemical additives to help create specific textures, colors, heat or light resistance, and flexibility.

Handle with Care

Despite the well-known durability of most plastic products, they will *always* have a small quantity of chemicals that are free to leach out under the right conditions. This is a problem because many of the building blocks used in plastics are highly toxic.

What's more, there are other dangerous chemical additives—including stabilizers, plasticizers, and colorants—that aren't part of the original polymer and can also leach out of the plastic and into our food, water, and soil.

Most of us learn when we're young that we're not allowed to throw a plastic bottle into the campfire even though it's cool to watch the plastic shrivel up and melt into liquid. If we do so, toxic gases—dioxins—are released and are extremely dangerous, especially if inhaled. Unfortunately, it's not very difficult to degrade your kitchen plasticware in the same way, whether or not you can see it or smell it happening.

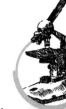

Cellular Truths

Toxic Communication

Many of the chemicals in plastic products have structural similarities to the hormones that provide communication throughout the human body, or they can bind to the steroid receptors on cell membranes and disrupt hormone actions. The same additives that provide flexibility, color, and flame retardant characteristics to plastic containers, for example, can migrate into food or water and have unintended effects on humans and animals.

"Environmental signaling" refers to the biological effects caused by chemicals in our environment that mimic natural hormones, and it's a rapidly developing hypothesis for how certain toxic elements in the environment are causing adverse health effects. Called *endocrine disruptors*, these chemicals can alter the body's hormone system and produce adverse developmental, reproductive, neurological, and immunological effects.

If this hypothesis is correct, then the victims are ourselves and our pets.

Developing fetuses and infants, whose neural and reproductive systems are still being formed, run the greatest risk of damage from endocrine disruptors. In laboratory studies, adverse consequences such as low fertility, premature sexual

Heating and microwaving, repeated washing with harsh detergents in dishwashers, scratching or cracking, and prolonged contact with fatty foods and oils will damage plastic enough to allow dangerous chemicals to leach out.

Wait, let's read that list again.

- Cleaning in the dishwasher
- Microwaving
- Storing with fatty or acidic foods

development, and cancer have been linked to early exposure to these hormone mimics.

These synthetic compounds are sending messages to us, but when our cells receive the information, they are confused and, as a result, cellular function is distorted.

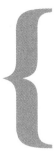

> Heating and microwaving, repeated washing with harsh detergents in dishwashers, scratching or cracking, and prolonged contact with fatty foods and oils will damage plastic enough to allow dangerous chemicals to leach out.

Those conveniences are what most people like about their plastic bowls, plates, cups, and containers! But the alternative is to wash all of your plasticware by hand, and never use it when warming up your food. So it's time to ask yourself: Why bother having it at all?

That's why my wife and I are methodically moving our kitchen to glass, which has none of the health issues inherent to plastic. In the interest of our health and the health of our child, we've purchased glass baby bottles, glass storage containers, and glass measuring cups, and we're doing away with plastic items that can degrade and leach toxins into our food.

Perilous Plastic

An entire series of books could be written on the many different forms of plastic and their potentially toxic elements. It would be impossible to sum up all of them here. However, there are a few commonly used plastic items you should avoid, *especially* when it comes to food preparation and storage in your kitchen.

Styrofoam Containers

Styrene—the building block for polystyrene—is described by the U.S. Environmental Protection Agency as a suspected carcinogen and a suspected toxin to the gastrointestinal, kidney, and respiratory systems.[16]

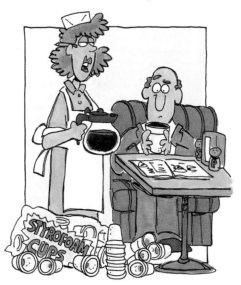

"Do you take styrene and ethylbenzene in your coffee?"

The foamed version of polystyrene is what we typically use to pack home restaurant leftovers. Polystyrene is also used for disposable cups, especially those made for hot drinks such as cocoa and coffee. Considering what we've just learned regarding heat and plastic, it won't come as a surprise to note that some studies have shown that chemicals leach from polystyrene when it's exposed to heat or oily substances.[17]

Yet most people use the "to go" container when they microwave their leftovers the next day and carry steaming hot coffee, tea, and cocoa in Styrofoam cups.

That's a scary thought.

The leaching of styrene may not even require heat, though. One study conducted by Louisiana State University showed that eggs—still in the shells—stored in Styrofoam containers for two weeks exhibited up to *seven times* more ethylbenzene and styrene than eggs fresh from the farm.[18] Those toxins are going right through the shells!

Despite this, many egg cartons are made with Styrofoam. (After reading the studies, I've opted to buy my eggs packaged in cardboard.)

To reduce our risk, my wife and I make it a habit to immediately transfer into a glass container any food we bring home from a restaurant. This way that fatty salmon or oily pasta isn't reacting with any plastic, and neither of us will be tempted to throw the styrofoam container into the microwave.

Baby Bottles and Water Bottles

As was mentioned at the beginning of this section, BPA is used in the manufacture of hard polycarbonate plastics, including baby bottles and reusable water bottles. You'll also find BPA in resins that line almost all food cans—from chicken noodle soup to green beans.

BPA is a potent endocrine disruptor that is known to mimic estrogen, and it has been shown to increase insulin resistance, chronic inflammation, and heart disease.[19]

Again, avoidance is your best bet. Although most baby bottle manufacturers in the United States have phased out BPA, it's still found in hard plastic (polycarbonate) water bottles. If you're unsure whether your water bottle is polycarbonate, look at the number in the middle of the recycling triangle stamped on the bottom. If it's a 7, it's likely BPA polycarbonate.

Getting rid of a polycarbonate water bottle is easy enough, and you can still drink plenty of liquids each day—as you should. Just make a stainless steel bottle your new best friend. You'll be able to take it everywhere for years before needing to replace it. If you're out shopping for a water bottle, don't opt for anything made from aluminum—these bottles are typically lined with BPA and will pose the same risks as polycarbonate bottles.

You should also avoid canned foods to reduce your risk from BPA. It may be impossible to rid your pantry of all canned foods, but at the very least try to avoid those for which you have fresh or frozen alternatives. Besides avoiding toxins, you'll also be getting more vitamins and minerals from unprocessed produce.

Manufacturers in Japan have already found a way to eliminate BPA from their canned foods, and I hope the United States can follow suit. As they have with BPA baby bottles, concerned consumers *must* motivate major food companies to act.

Plastic Wrap

For years the plastic wrap you would place around your baked goods and leftovers was made from polyvinyl chloride (PVC).

PVC is a hard, resinous material that requires plasticizers, stabilizers, flame retardants, and lubricants to be of any practical value. These additives—which aren't chemically bonded to the plastic's basic building blocks—are what make PVC one of the most toxic plastics in our homes today.

One such additive, phthalic acid, is often used in PVC to increase pliability. As we learned earlier, phthalates have numerous adverse health effects, including metabolism interference, thyroid dysfunction, early puberty, and allergies. One of the most consistent reports concerns reproductive impairment of young boys, and this result likely occurs in the womb. When a pregnant woman is exposed to phthalates—whether from plastic or personal-care products—this harmful chemical can cross the placenta and enter fetal circulation. Problems for boys exposed to phthalates in this manner may include depleted male hormone levels, undescended testes, decreased fertility, and an increased risk of testicular cancer.[20]

You read that correctly: It's possible that an infant boy who is exposed to phthalates while in his mother's womb could feel the effects twenty or thirty years later with testicular cancer.

> It's possible that an infant boy who is exposed to phthalates while in his mother's womb could feel the effects twenty or thirty years later with testicular cancer.

Due to consumer concerns about phthalates, most major manufacturers have begun using a different plastic—low-density polyethylene (LDPE)—to make plastic-wrap products for regular home use. Although LDPE-based plastic wrap doesn't contain phthalates, it's less effective than wrap made from PVC at clinging to packaging and sealing in odors. (You may have noticed this yourself and wondered what had changed.)

Thus, most delis, butchers, caterers, and restaurants continue to use PVC-based wrap.

Fortunately, it's not that hard to reduce your exposure to PVC, even from deli and grocery store packaging. *National Geographic's* "Green Guide" gives this advice: Unwrap your product when you get home from the grocery store. If possible, trim away any meat or cheese that was touching the PVC wrap or Styrofoam tray, and then store it in a glass container that seals with a lid.[21]

Simple Solution:
If you use plastic wrap, ensure it's **LDPE**-based plastic, and regardless of what type it is, never use it in the microwave.

The Plastic Code

Plastics are categorized based on their chemical makeup and the extent to which they can be recycled. By learning to recognize the symbols and numbers on the bottom of your plastic purchases, you can make better choices for you and your family. These numbers appear in a triangular symbol that looks like this.

01 (PET): Polyethylene terephthalate is used in high-impact packaging, water and soft drink bottles, cooking oil containers, and microwave food trays. **Considered safe under normal conditions but will degrade over time.**

02 (PE-HD/HDPE): High-density polyethylene, the more durable form of PET, is used for opaque or cloudy containers that hold personal-care products, vitamins, detergents, milk jugs, and motor oil. Not appropriate for hot liquids. **It's considered safe under normal conditions but will degrade over time.**

03 (PVC): Polyvinyl chloride is found in shower curtains, meat and cheese wrappers, binders, some shrink wrap, plumbing materials, vinyl flooring, and much, much more. Contains highly toxic phthalate plasticizers that can leach into food or beverages. **Avoid whenever and wherever possible, especially in the kitchen.**

04 (PE-LD/LDPE): Low-density polyethylene is used in shopping bags, CD cases, computers, most consumer shrink wrap, and product packaging. **It's generally considered safe.**

05 (PP):   Polypropylene is found in bottle caps, diapers, lots of kitchenware, yogurt and cottage cheese containers, and electronic product packaging. **Heat-resistant, reusable, and considered the safest plastic for human use.**

06 (PS):   Polystyrene is used in take-out food containers, drinking cups, egg cartons, and building materials. Composed of possible human carcinogens. **Known to degrade and leach toxins when exposed to high heat or oil; avoid whenever and wherever possible.**

07 (O):   All other plastics not listed above are placed in this "other" category, as indicated by the "O," including polycarbonate, polyurethane, acrylic, fiberglass, nylon, and more environmentally friendly hybrid plastics. **Many are considered safe, but be aware that polycarbonate bottles that contain BPA are considered part of this group.**

These are the key pieces of information you should take away from this chart:

- The safest plastics to use (and reuse) are denoted with the number 5 (PP).
- Plastics in the 1 (PET), 2 (PE-HD), and 4 (PE-LD) categories are generally safe, but have some issues with toxicity and a limited shelf life.
- Avoid products labeled 3 (PVC), 6 (PS), and 7 (O) in regard to food or liquid packaging (unless you know for certain the number 7 plastic is a special biodegradable hybrid).

Though this book is focused on the smaller stage of the home, it's important to remember that plastic has an impact on our much larger world.

Most plastic is made from nonrenewable resources such as crude oil. That alone should give us pause because it's a nonrenewable resource upon which so much depends. But even if we had access to unlimited petroleum, we would still need to recognize that the same properties that make plastic so incredible—relative durability and chemical stability—can also make plastic a major threat to our environment.

If not recycled or disposed of properly, plastic ends up in our waterways, degrading so slowly that there are now massive "plastic islands" floating in the Pacific and Atlantic oceans. Bit by bit, lighters, trinkets, grocery bags, and containers break into smaller fragments that fish, marine mammals, and seabirds mistake for food.[22] This can be a lethal mistake—both for the animals and for us.

Suddenly, the toxins we've worked so hard to avoid in our home are found in the marine food chain, where they will make their way back to our dinner tables.

By making some of the small changes that we've discussed in these pages, such as recycling plastic whenever possible and encouraging those around you to do the same, you can make a positive difference in your health and the health of our world.

Simple Solution:

Purchase reusable grocery bags made of natural materials such as cotton and use them as often as you can.

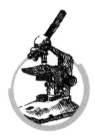

Chapter 9
Drink Up!

We can't talk about the health aspects of our food without considering the drinks we use to wash it all down.

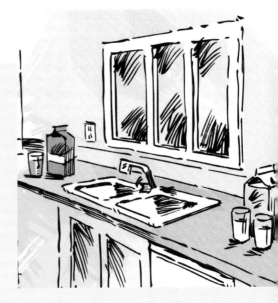

In a society in which people consume an average of 450 calories a day just from beverages—nearly twice as many as thirty years ago[1]— the beverages we consume with our meals are taking on increasing importance. Even those of us who choose water most of the time may face serious risks. It's time to consider whether our "cup runneth over" with life-giving liquid, empty calories, or— worst of all—poisons.

QUIZ **How Toxic Is Your Home?**   Scores

1. Is milk your main source of calcium? Yes_____ (8 pts)

2. Which of the following beverages do you often consume? (Select all that apply)
   ☐ Store-bought fruit drinks/cocktails (8 pts)   ☐ Home-squeezed juice (0 pts)
   ☐ Store-bought 100 percent juice (4 pts)   ☐ I don't drink my fruit (0 pts)

3. Is your home water fluoridated? Yes_____ (10 pts)

4. How many beverages, including water, do you consume at a typical meal?

No liquids	Small Drink	Large Drink	X-Large Drink	Refills
0 pts	2 pts	5 pts	8 pts	12 pts

5. How many caffeinated beverages do you consume each day? Count those "extra large," "grande," and "super-big" beverages as two or more drinks. (4 pts each)

Your "Drink" danger score

1–12	13–24	25–36	37+
Hydrated	Getting thirsty	Parched	Bone-dry

Water Wasteland

It's ironic that the two most critical ingredients that create and sustain all life on earth—oxygen and water—are taken for granted as things to which we are entitled. We've been taught that the best things in life are free and, accordingly, we treat air and water as if they will be prefiltered constantly and automatically by natural forces to maintain the quality required for us to live and grow.

In chapter 3, we discussed the importance of focusing on air quality in every room of the home—especially in the bedrooms, where much of our time is spent to replenish, repair, and renew our cells during sleep. Most of us are aware of the thousands of pollutants released into the atmosphere by our factories, power plants, and vehicles, and we are routinely notified by our TV weather commentators regarding the air quality or lack thereof for the coming week.

Air pollution, "the greenhouse effect," and global warming dominate the primetime news. However, we almost never hear about the elixir of life itself: our water supply.

A Trace Too Much

As alarming as many scientists find the levels of toxic chemicals and pollutants in our water supply to be, we consumers are mostly oblivious to the fact that our families are slowly being poisoned.

If water looks clean coming out of the tap, we assume it must be safe. The amounts of toxins may be small, but we need to drink as much water as we can to be healthy. It's the ultimate paradox: With every life-giving sip, we accumulate more and more of the bad stuff in our systems.

Just like slow weight gain—that creep of just one or two pounds a year—subtle poisoning from our water supply will rarely gain our notice until we suddenly and very personally feel the effects. We need a wake-up call and a direct approach to avoid what's unacceptable in our water while taking positive action to protect ourselves.

How many of us are concerned about drinking water when we go camping or when we travel, but don't give it a second thought in our own homes?

It might change your mind to know that the Safe Drinking Water Act of 1974 covers only ninety-one contaminants, yet an estimated *60,000 chemicals* are used within the United States.[2] Make no mistake: Many of those chemicals find their way into our streams, rivers, lakes, and, ultimately, into our water supplies. According to an article appearing in the *New York Times* on December 7, 2009, the newspaper's own research—conducted since 2004—found that the water provided to more than 49 million people had contained illegal concentrations of chemicals such as arsenic or radioactive substances such as uranium as well as dangerous bacteria often found in sewage.[3]

{ The Safe Drinking Water Act of 1974 covers only ninety-one contaminants, yet an estimated *60,000 chemicals* are used within the United States. }

Power plants are a major source of toxic by-products. Much of that waste once went into the atmosphere, but because of stricter air pollution laws, it now more often goes into rivers, lakes, or landfills that leach into nearby groundwater.

Agricultural runoff is the single biggest contributor to water pollution in rivers and streams, according to the EPA. However, farm waste is largely unregulated by many of the federal laws designed to prevent pollution and protect drinking water supplies. As rainwater runoff washes over our grassy areas, it picks up residuals from the 67 million pounds of fertilizer and pesticides we apply each year and deposits them in our surface water and groundwater.

As we have become a modern industrial society with a huge population migration moving people from rural to urban communities, our sewer systems have become inadequate to meet the growing demand, leading to sewage spilling into our waterways and polluting them with human and animal waste as well as industrial chemicals. When I was a student living in San Diego we often had warnings not to go swimming in the ocean due to sewage contamination.

This discussion isn't meant to be a scare tactic for shock effect. The goal here is awareness so that we can be proactive in making the home an oasis for our families to enjoy the best quality of life possible.

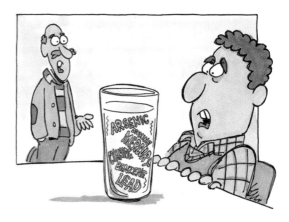

"What, do you have a bug in your water?"

"I wish."

The Fluoride Fairy Tale

One of the main contaminants in tap water is something our local government often adds on purpose. We covered some of the dangers fluoride poses in chapter 5 in the discussion about toothpaste.

However, much of our water supply also contains fluoride, coming either from natural sources or having been put there by a local water district. A study requested by the EPA and recently issued by the National Research Council reported that "the high levels of fluoride that occur naturally in some drinking water can cause tooth and bone damage, and should be reduced."[4] Other studies have found that sodium fluoride can compromise cellular health and result in adverse thyroid function and adverse neurological effects. Unfortunately, according to the study, artificially fluoridated water flows into the homes of more than 160 million Americans.[5]

What many people *don't* realize is that silicofluorides—the chemicals used to artificially fluoridate a water supply—are in essence industrial waste from phosphate mining and manufacturing. This means the fertilizer industry gets to offload its toxic waste to water districts around the country and do so as a "public health" product! It's baffling to realize that fluorine gas compounds are regulated as serious pollutants in our air but can be converted into a supposedly beneficial additive to our water.

The story of fluoridated water may have an even darker angle than corporate greed. There have long been rumors that Nazi Germany employed fluoridated water for its potential neurotoxic effects. Fluoride was theorized to make people more docile and easy to control, and thus it was added to water supplies in occupied regions and POW camps. We'll let the online forums continue to debate whether this is a myth or historical fact, but it's an excellent example of how little we really know about the safety of the chemicals found in our everyday products and services.

We're not just getting fluoride from our tap water and tooth brushing, either. Bottled water often contains fluoride, as do sodas, juices, and many foods manufactured using artificially fluoridated water. Between all of these sources, you can easily exceed the recommended dose

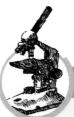

Cellular Truths

Too Much Fluoride

Fluorine, better known as fluoride, is the most electronegative and reactive of all the elements. It binds tenaciously to other elements and compounds, preventing them from entering into other chemical reactions. The presence of just one fluoride atom in any size molecule can totally change its nature and function. Fluoride has the ability to poison even the strongest of the body's enzyme systems.

Most importantly, fluoride—as with mercury, antimony, and arsenic—inhibits the Krebs cycle that produces the ATP energy required for powering all cellular functions.

Body accumulations of fluoride from exposure through the mouth, our respiratory tract, or skin are greatest in the calcified tissues of the skeleton or teeth. In humans, these tissues undergo remodeling throughout life. Cells called osteoclasts steadily dismantle tissue in bones and other cells called osteoblasts assemble new tissue to replace the old. Collagen, the main protein in connective tissue, is an organic matrix for the deposition of the minerals calcium and phosphorus. When fluoride ions are incorporated into the matrix instead, the mineralization profile shifts to higher densities and hardness. It is thought that the wider fluoride crystals do not associate with the collagen matrix as well as calcium.

of daily fluoride consumption and start to see negative health effects. For this reason, even the pro-fluoride American Dental Association recommends that infant formula be mixed with nonfluoridated water to make certain bottle-fed babies don't receive toxic levels of fluoride.[6]

Distilled water, which can be purchased in most grocery stores, is likely the best choice for infants and young children who live in areas where tap water is fluoridated. Distilled water may lack the beneficial minerals found in some water supplies, but it will also be free of many common impurities, like fluoride, that could harm children's more vulnerable bodies.

Most countries in modern-day Western Europe have opted out of artificially fluoridated water, dismissing the practice for what it really is: mass medication. This moderate approach to the issue allows individuals to choose whether they—and their children—want fluoride.

The one-size-fits-all remedy suggested for dental health is not the answer.

What You Can Do

Knowing what we do about water contamination, it's no surprise that bottled water is now a $4 billion-a-year business in the United States, with millions of us willing to pay 240 to 10,000 times more per gallon

This results in greater bone brittleness and reduced mechanical strength, which increases the risk of bone fractures, especially in the elderly. Incidence of hip fractures continues to increase in the United States, and too often these fractures initiate a cascade of complications that end in death.

Many studies have shown the effects of fluoride on bones and teeth to be biphasic. That is, small amounts of fluoride can make bones stronger, but over a certain threshold the effects become negative, resulting in weaker, more brittle bones. At higher concentrations fluoride is mitogenic to osteoblasts and toxic to osteoclasts. Its effect on blast cells is to stimulate cellular proliferation, with possible development of osteosarcoma, a cancerous bone tumor.

Moderate to high fluoride exposure in children may result in dental fluorosis. Fluorosis begins with small white striations across teeth, but can progress to discolored, pitted teeth that are subject to fracture.

In addition to bone brittleness and skeletal and dental fluorosis, fluoride damage due to molecular displacement extends to cells of the brain, liver, kidney, lungs, gastrointestinal tract, blood vessels, skin, and thyroid. For example, the critical role of thyroid hormone in regulating the metabolism of every cell in the body is disrupted when fluoride displaces iodine, resulting in hypothyroidism—which can lead to constipation, depression, fatigue, weight gain, joint and muscle pain, and much more.

for bottled water than we do for tap water. But bottled water isn't necessarily less contaminated than tap water. In fact, about a quarter of bottled water is simply tap water in a bottle.[7] Although required to meet the same safety standards as public water supplies, bottled water does not undergo the same testing and reporting as water from a treatment facility. Water that is bottled and sold in the same state may not be subject to any federal standards at all.

And bottled water is at risk of contamination from the plasticizers and other chemicals that make up the plastic bottle it is stored in. Ironically, if those billions of bottles aren't disposed of properly, they can go on to contaminate the very water that will be used to fill new bottles.

If you frequently drink bottled water, never reuse your bottle, especially if it has become worn or scratched. This damages the plastic's integrity and increases the leaching of harmful chemicals into your life-giving water. And if you let your plastic water bottle sit out in a hot car or somewhere else that heats the water and plastic, you have greatly increased the chemicals leaching into your water and should immediately and properly dispose of the bottle— even if it's full. All the stuff that's in our water to start with is bad enough; don't make it worse by handling the containers poorly.

The simplest solution? Make a stainless steel water bottle—filled with purified water—your new companion.

Home Treatment Systems

If you want a safe water supply at home and wish to avoid the financial and environmental burden of bottled water, you can install either "point-of-entry" (POE) systems, which treat all the water entering the house, or simply add "point-of-use" (POU) systems, which treat water at a single tap. Point-of-use systems are usually located under a sink, on a counter top, or on the faucet itself.

Activated Carbon Filtration:

These replaceable cartridges containing granular carbon help remove pesticides, solvents, lead, chlorine, some heavy metals, and some microbes. The filters are typically located in a portable pitcher, under the sink, or on the faucet. Although carbon filters are a good, inexpensive place to start with in-home water filtration, they do not remove fluoride, all heavy metals, and other contaminants. Reverse osmosis and distillation are more comprehensive solutions for ensuring that you have clean, healthy tap water.

Simple Solution:

Use a pitcher with an activated carbon filter to reduce contaminants in your water. Although it won't filter out all pollutants, it's a good start at a low cost.

Reverse Osmosis:

Found on the counter top or under the sink, this filtration method removes fluoride, nitrate, bacteria, pesticides, solvents, lead, and foul tastes by moving water through a thin membrane, trapping contaminants on the other side. Many in-home reverse osmosis systems also use activated carbon filtration.

Distillation:

This process removes impurities like bacteria, nitrates, sodium, and many organic compounds by boiling water into steam, which then condenses into a clean container. Distillation systems can be wall-mounted or located on a countertop.

For more information on treatment systems, visit www.myhealthyhome.com/water.

Water truly is the elixir of life.

It constitutes more than 70 percent of solid body tissue and helps regulate body temperature, carry nutrients and oxygen to our cells, remove waste, cushion joints, and protect organs and tissues. Although most of us understand that we should drink sixty-four fluid ounces of water daily, we're often in various stages of dehydration because we either drink less than half the water we need or consume too many alternative water-robbing beverages.

We think we're doing fine by substituting milk, juice, coffee, and soft drinks in our daily routines, not realizing that we regularly overdose on caffeinated or alcoholic beverages that are diuretics, which dehydrate us by causing the body to lose water through increased urination. If you are consuming these "undrinks," you need to drink additional water to compensate.

Simple Solution:
Don't forget to drink as much water in cold weather as you do when summer arrives.

Water is one case in which quantity is probably even more important than quality. If your choice is between being dehydrated or drinking unpurified tap water, pick the tap water. I often struggle when I'm staying in a hotel and don't have any purified water. But it's always better to risk the tap water than suffer the known adverse effects of dehydration, which will *definitely* damage my cells.

The bottom line is this: Make your home water supply as safe as possible and drink those eight glasses of water every day. Don't wait until you are thirsty. Your body needs that precious stuff that constitutes life.

A Final Word about Water

Although we've highlighted the many long-term health concerns that our modern water supply poses, these issues pale in comparison to the serious drought and appalling water contamination that millions in third-world countries face. In the United States and Canada, we're able to indulge in what are likely some of the world's best water supplies, which can then easily be improved by individuals in their very own home.

If in the course of eliminating plastic from your kitchen, you've made the commitment to stop purchasing bottled water, please consider donating what you would have spent each month on this usually unnecessary consumable to a charity that helps provide clean water to people in less fortunate regions.

You can find links to great charities on our Web site, www.myhealthyhome.com/charity.

All the Wrong Drinks for All the Wrong Reasons

It's not just our water that should be scrutinized under a microscope. Our beverage choices abound, and all of them should be addressed—whether they deserve room in our refrigerator and why they *don't* deserve room at the dining table.

The Short on Soda

We all know soda's bad for us. The sugar, the calories, the caffeine, the acid, the high-fructose corn syrup, the artificial sweeteners. Yet many of us stop by our local convenience store every day and get a *big* plastic cup full of the stuff. We could cite numerous studies and statistics here about why we should avoid soda, but most of it wouldn't be new or surprising.

In short, we're exchanging the life-giving properties of water for the empty calories and dehydration of cola.

This is one of the simplest solutions in the book: Don't drink soda.

You may need to wean yourself off it, slowly replacing one Big Gulp® at a time with water, but you'll see a difference—in your skin, your hair, your waistline, and your overall health.

Myths about Milk

Since we were old enough to understand what Mom was saying, we've been taught how important it is to drink our milk at each meal so we would have strong teeth and bones. The calcium in the milk is what made our bones healthy enough to support our body when we ran and jumped.

Mom was right. Calcium *is* important. However, there's no good evidence that consuming more than one serving of milk per day will reduce fracture risk. Milk isn't the only—or even a good—source of calcium. Only in recent years has consumption of cow's milk been identified as a nutritional concern. Only since humans developed refrigeration have we been able to put milk on the table every day—not only for children, but for adults as well, for as long as they live. Even today, for most of the world's populations, drinking milk after the age of three or four simply isn't part of a normal diet.

When we say that everyone should drink milk or consume dairy products in order to obtain enough calcium for strong bones, we're forgetting that 90 percent of Asians, 70 percent of blacks and Native Americans, and 50 percent of Hispanics are lactose intolerant—they can't digest milk, and when they drink it they may suffer severe gastrointestinal symptoms. Yet these people aren't plagued by rickets and osteoporosis.

How do they do it?

Even those who *are* able to consume dairy products should consider the fact that whole milk is high in saturated fats, which pose a risk factor for heart disease. High levels of galactose, a sugar that's released by the digestion of lactose in milk, have been associated with increased risk of ovarian cancer. In a Harvard study of health professionals, men who drank two or more glasses of milk a day were almost twice as likely to develop advanced prostate cancer as those who didn't drink milk at all.[8]

Finally, whole milk contains high levels of protein, which increases calcium excretion in the urine. In the process of metabolizing protein, our bodies produce phosphoric and sulfuric acids. These acids must be buffered with calcium, which is drawn out of the bones. The calcium is bound to the acids and lost during excretion. So even though milk does provide some calcium, it cancels out its benefits by being acid-producing and drawing calcium from your bones.

You can reduce calcium loss by increasing intake of alkalizing vegetables, which are major sources of calcium in themselves.[9] A reasonable diet typically provides about 300 mg of calcium per day from nondairy sources.

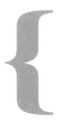

> Even though milk does provide some calcium, it cancels out its benefits by being acid-producing and drawing calcium from your bones.

And there are many other nutrients that influence bone health, some of which may be more deserving of attention than calcium. One source indicates that there are "at least" eighteen nutrients essential for healthy bones.[10] They include minerals, such as calcium, of course, magnesium, and phosphorus; vitamins, such as C, D, and K; and other nutrients like essential fatty acids and protein. Shortages of any of these nutrients can inhibit calcium absorption or incorporation into the bone structure.

Though a majority of Americans are calcium deficient, it isn't difficult to boost your calcium intake, either through diet or supplementation.[11]

In the United States and many other industrialized countries, osteoporosis—the thinning of bone tissue and loss of bone density that takes place over time—isn't as much a result of inadequate calcium intake as it is a matter of calcium *loss*. This loss is

Simple Solution:
Weight lifting exercises are one of the best ways to improve your bone density.

due to all the factors noted above. Plenty of exercise, a nourishing diet, and an otherwise healthy lifestyle can all contribute to healthy bones and teeth. Milk consumption isn't a factor—no matter *what* Mom said.

Fresh-Squeezed

We learned in the previous chapter that the more fruits and vegetables are "prepared," or processed, the more likely they will lose valuable nutrients. So it should come as no surprise that fruit juices typically aren't the best sources when it comes to getting vitamins and antioxidants. A recent study by the University of Arizona found that when store-bought orange juice—in a carton—is opened, the already diminished vitamin C levels rapidly deteriorate. After a few weeks in your refrigerator, your orange juice may not contain *any* vitamin C![12]

Most fruit juices you buy in the grocery store—even 100 percent juices with no added sugar—are simply high-glycemic, high-calorie snacks. And "juice drinks" or "juice cocktails" seem to have everything *but* fruit juice in them. Just take a look at the label—water, high-fructose corn syrup, flavorings, and a tiny squeeze of whatever fruit the manufacturer wants to display on the label. These fruit drinks amount to little more than juicy sodas and aren't worth the added calories or rapid rise in the blood sugar—*especially* for our children. I'm proud to say that our son doesn't drink juice. He gets his nourishment from food and his hydration from water filtered by reverse osmosis.

Simple Solution:

If you love juice, make your own natural juices at home to receive the benefits of fruit pulp, fruit skin, and even vegetables.

When we're craving the deliciousness of a ripe red apple, we should eat an apple, not drink it. The skin and pulp contain life-giving carotenoids, flavonoids, and fiber, which help lower the glycemic load of naturally sugary fruit.

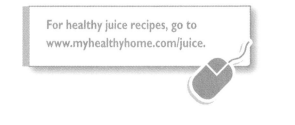

For healthy juice recipes, go to www.myhealthyhome.com/juice.

Washing It Down

Regardless of what your favorite beverage is, remember that it should be consumed away from the table. Dr. Wentz has confused many a waiter by refusing the glass of water that's offered before meals. A few poor souls have made the mistake of asking why. His answer is, in essence, that the stomach was meant to be acidic and full of enzymes to digest your foods. When you dilute that environment with a gallon of soda or a half-gallon of water, your waterlogged digestive system is rendered less effective.

Thus, your colorful, organic, fresh, low-glycemic vegetables are largely intact when they're passing through you. So how can you get any nutrients from them? This problem is even more profound with children, who can fill their small stomachs with the contents of their juice bottles. Not only are they not absorbing food nutrients, they're not eating much food at all.

Few things have done more to damage our nutritional intake than the super-duper-sized drink. If you must wash your food down with a beverage, limit the volume as much as possible. Stop flushing your nutrients through your system and down the toilet—drink the majority of your beverages in between meals.

Simple Solutions Summary

As important as it is to eliminate hidden dangers throughout our home, the easiest place to make a significant difference in our lifelong health is in the kitchen. Without proper fuel and hydration, our body cannot hope to mount a defense against an increasingly toxic world.

Yet too many of us are consuming the equivalent of dietary refuse—food and beverages that contain sickening ingredients, lack life-giving nutrients, and are prepared and delivered using toxic methods. The plethora of choices that must be made in our kitchens may seem downright disheartening at times, yet with a few changes, that room can become a refuge of abundant nutrition, delicious flavors, and revitalizing conversation.

What Simple Solutions will you add to your Kitchen?

Scores

1. I will: (Select all that apply)

- ☐ Cut consumption of high-glycemic "white" foods like white bread, white rice, and potatoes in half (10 pts)
- ☐ Add more brightly colored fruits and vegetables to my diet each day (2 pts per additional daily serving)
- ☐ Switch from one daily high-glycemic snack like potato chips to a low-glycemic snack like almonds (2 pts)
- ☐ Replace white flour with whole, multi-grain flour (5 pts)
- ☐ Serve one meal a day that consists of 60–80 percent alkalizing fruits and vegetables (8 pts)

2. I will: (Select all that apply)

- ☐ Eliminate processed, high-sodium foods like condensed soups, frozen meals, and cured meats from my diet (3 pts for each food regularly eaten)
- ☐ Add more potassium-rich food sources to my daily diet (3 pts for each)
- ☐ Trade in regular table salt for natural sea salt (2 pts)
- ☐ Drink a glass of lemon water every morning (3 pts)
- ☐ Throw out any trans-fats in the refrigerator or cupboards and replace them with extra virgin olive oil, canola oil, or grape seed oil (8 pts)

3. I will: (Select all that apply)

- ☐ Switch from boiling vegetables to steaming them (5 pts)
- ☐ Eliminate unnecessary chopping and slicing of fresh vegetables (3 pts)
- ☐ Maintain a safe distance (at least five feet) from the microwave when it's running (4 pts)
- ☐ Stop grilling meat (5 pts) or reduce the heat on the grill (2 pts) to reduce charring
- ☐ Trade in nonstick cookware for pans that are free of Teflon (PTFE) (2 pts for each pan)
- ☐ If keeping nonstick cookware, use only medium or lower heat (2 pts)

4. I will: (Select all that apply)

- ☐ Switch my plastic/foam containers to glass (10 pts)
- ☐ If keeping plastic kitchenware, stop putting it in the microwave (6 pts) and/or dishwasher (4 pts)
- ☐ Stop using plastic wrap in the kitchen (8 pts)
- ☐ Remove restaurant leftovers from plastic/foam containers as soon as I get home (3 pts)

5. I will: (Select one)

   ☐ Install a reverse osmosis water purification device in the kitchen (15 pts)

   ☐ Use an inexpensive pitcher filter to eliminate some tap water contaminants (8 pts)

   ☐ At the very least, give infants and small children distilled water if the tap water is fluoridated (3 pts)

6. I will: (Select all that apply)

   ☐ Drink at least 64 oz. of purified water each day (6 pts)

   ☐ Trade in plastic bottled water for filtered tap water in a reusable stainless steel bottle (5 pts)

7. I will: (Select all that apply)

   ☐ Stop drinking soda, whether it's diet or not (8 pts)

   ☐ Cut out processed juices and "juice drinks" for the family (5 pts)

   ☐ Make juice with a juicer/blender and include the pulp and skins (2 pts)

   ☐ Reduce milk consumption (3 pts)

   ☐ Cut back on water/drinks with meals (6 pts for no beverages; 4 pts for small drinks)

Your Simple Solutions positive score:	
Your "Food" danger score:	-
Your "Cooking" danger score:	-
Your "Drink" danger score:	-
Your Kitchen Health total:	

Are you making a positive difference?

You can track your quiz scores and solution points on *The Healthy Home* Web site at www.myhealthyhome.com. Be sure to get your Web access code in the back of the book.

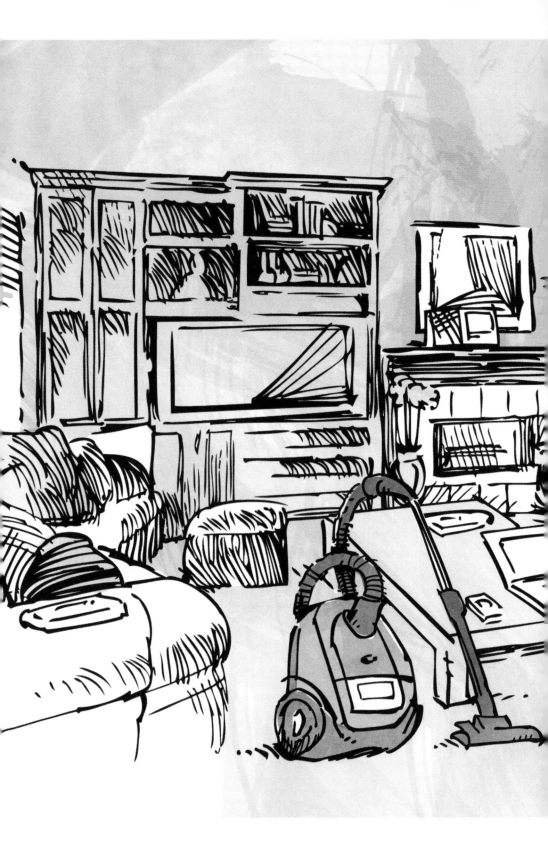

5

Living Areas

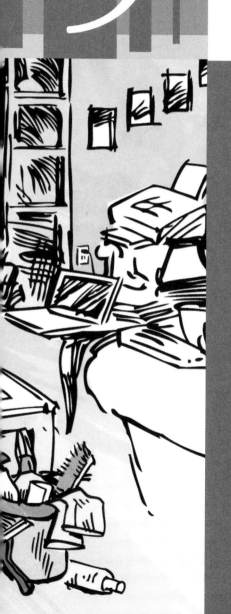

Living areas should be just that, places where we *live*. Good friends and family share these refuges where we unwind at the end of the day. Often we keep them cleaned, polished, shiny, and inviting with the fresh-smelling magic-in-a-can. Recliners, throws, books, and fireplaces share the space with large-screen TVs, sound systems, video games, and home office equipment.

They're all wonderful gadgets, but they can quickly turn our living space into a dead zone, where the only real interaction is between our brains and competing electromagnetic fields. We must pay particular attention to our living areas so we don't pollute our bodies, minds, or relationships.

Having spent time chatting around the island in the kitchen, we follow Dave into a comfortable, contemporary living room. The furniture, positioned to make conversation easy, is upholstered in warm, textured neutrals that are offset by brightly colored throw pillows and a rich, brown wool rug. A fireplace flanked by built-in bookshelves beckons the visitor to curl up on the couch for a good read, although the impressive home theater system is tempting, too. The personal photographs that adorn the walls are the final touch for making this room a relaxing gathering place for friends and family.

Around a corner, steps lead to a second-floor landing, and over a low wall, the edge of a computer screen is visible and reveals an open office.

Dave: We were intentional with the material we chose for the décor. We picked materials that are easy to maintain so we don't have to rely on heavy cleaners. We also tried to use natural wood glues and finishes, but we still have some work to do.

Donna: What sort of things did you need to consider in relation to the baby?

Dave: Reneé has done a ton of research on making this a safe place for Andrew. He's toddling all over the place, gumming the couch cushions and chewing on anything he can get hold of.

Donna: Given the concerns you have for chemical cleaners, what's used on these floors to keep them so shiny?

Dave: To be perfectly honest, I don't do the floors very often, but I do know Reneé has experimented with old-school cleaner recipes like baking soda and vinegar. She's been pretty happy with the results. We haven't gone *totally* low tech, though. We use our steam mop all the time.

Dr. Wentz: It's amazing how things come full circle. The cleaning industry has spent the past three decades creating products for cleaning jobs that we didn't even know we wanted to do, and now we're looking back at what our mothers or grandmothers used to scrub their floors.

Donna: The old-school attitude about dirt was different, as well. It was assumed that kids are tough and resilient and that a little dirt won't hurt.

Dr. Wentz: In fact, good, unpolluted dirt is actually good for kids. It's the "chemical clean" that worries me, along with fire retardants. Our air is actually full of contaminants. We err in thinking that if we can't see it, there's nothing there. It's those microscopic contaminants we need to be concerned about. *[He pulls out his Gauss meter.]* That, and the Wi-Fi that permeates every foot of living space. When I get close to the office landing the meter is going crazy. *[He glances at Dave.]*

Dave: Guilty as charged. Although I love gadgets, I put most of the home entertainment and technology systems in the office to keep them away from areas Andrew would be playing in. The central control system puts out some EMFs, but we don't sit too close to it, and we keep Andrew out of there as much as possible. Children are more susceptible to the dangers.

Dr. Wentz: We must be mindful of technology for many reasons. Our days and tasks run together, so we are as busy at night as we are in the day. There's value to disengaging ourselves from our electronic attachments, setting boundaries around work and play, and nurturing our most important relationships.

Dave: *[Laughs.]* This from the man who still dictates most of his research. You need to *engage* in technology before you can disengage, Dad.

Donna: Given your career, Dave, how have you managed to set any such boundaries?

Dave: It's definitely been a struggle at times. But I learned pretty quickly this past year that if I didn't disconnect from my e-mail and phone in the evening, I'd miss out on a lot of important firsts with Andrew. It's been great spending more time with my family.

Chapter 10
Clean Living

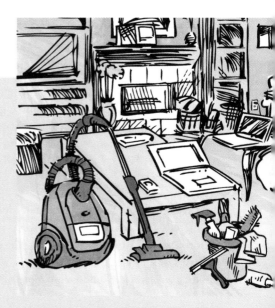

Despite increasingly frantic schedules, we spend a huge percentage of our lives at home. For most of us, it's a haven from the outside world. And because of that, we harbor some illusions that can be dangerous.

Beyond the walls of our homes, we are well aware of dangers such as air pollution and industrial waste, and we feel safe and cozy behind our tightly sealed windows and doors. Yet just like in the scary movies we all watched as kids, the killer we think is "out there" is really locked inside the house with us.

QUIZ How Toxic Is Your Home?   Scores

1. What does your house smell like when it's been cleaned?		
Nothing	Scented cleaners	Bleach/ammonia
0 pts	6 pts	12 pts

2. Do you wear gloves when you clean? No_____ (8 pts)

3. Do you wear your shoes in the house? Yes_____ (8 pts)

4. How often do you use air/fabric fresheners?			
Never	Monthly	Weekly	Daily
0 pts	2 pts	6 pts	10 pts

Your "Clean" danger score

1–7	8–14	15–21	22+
Next to godliness	Needs a dusting	Quite a mess	Living in squalor

Fight for Your Environment

Indoor air pollution is one of the enemies our bodies must contend with day and night. We look outside and think the air is polluted, but we don't stop to think about where our home's air comes from.

In modern homes—which often are sealed as tightly as Tupperware®—the low level of pollution from outside air is pumped inside and concentrated with the fumes from the hundreds of products we use inside, thus creating a seriously nasty indoor atmosphere. As mentioned in chapter 3, the air we're breathing while indoors is usually two to five times more polluted than outdoor air with all of its organic pollutants.[1]

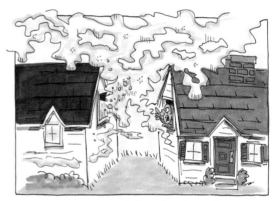

It was a 'good air quality' day until Mrs. Jones opened her window.

The cumulative effect of pollutants in our living areas ought to be a grave concern. Toxic glue holds down our synthetic pads and carpet. The paint on our walls is emitting gasses. Our furniture is sprayed with fire-retardant, stain-resistant chemicals, and dyed with even more chemicals. The many chemical fragrances from our hygiene and cleaning products are wafting through the house.

But don't pull out the gas mask just yet.

Take one simple step to make a huge difference—open the windows! In doing so you just saved your family from *millions* of contaminants floating around in your air, and it didn't cost a thing.

Many safe and efficient options are now available for sprucing up the air

Simple Solution:
Open your windows—often.

inside your home. When it does come time to build or remodel, take the time to educate yourself about the components you are using. There are low-VOC paints and natural carpets. You can also ask for less toxic glues and materials. But for now, start by airing out your house and breathing easier.

Time to Repaint?

Is your house paint looking dull and smudged? A can of paint can go a long way toward changing the mood of a room. We chose deep reds to complement shades of white, gray, and cream as we set out to transform our loft. Fortunately, the latest in wall coatings will provide plenty of style yet give off lower emissions.

Paints labeled eco-friendly are generally manufactured to contain fewer volatile organic compounds (VOCs). When buying an interior paint, look for products containing 50 grams or less per liter of VOCs for a flat paint, and 150 grams or less per liter for a gloss paint. Quality paint manufacturers will list the VOC grams per liter right on the paint can or in their sales literature at the store. If you can't find the listing, ask a customer service representative for assistance. Another indication that the paint has met high-performance and tight emissions standards is the EcoLogo seal, or the symbol of a similar eco-certification program such as Green Seal.

See the Light

When most people buy a light bulb, they think about watts, price, energy savings, appearance, and the expected life of the bulb. But two additional factors should be considered when purchasing light bulbs, as they could have a direct impact on our health.

First, what is the light spectrum of the bulb? Most fluorescent light bulbs only give one spectrum of light and can leave you feeling drained and lethargic. They actually suck the life out of you and everyone else who is subjected to them, whether at the office or mall. So don't bring them home with you!

Second, how is the light produced? Most governments and environmental groups are "putting on the heavy" to save energy by switching to CFLs—Compact Fluorescent Lights. The difference between a CFL and regular incandescent bulb is that CFLs typically have a spiral shape and cost more due to their longer life and energy-saving qualities. Those qualities may sound wonderful, but CFLs also typically provide unhealthy, harsh light, and they are *extremely* dangerous if they break.

Let's face it, all light bulbs break, whether it's in your home or somewhere along the way to the landfill. And when these little vessels of death break, they release one of the most toxic gases known to man—mercury vapor. Read the instructions on a CFL box about the disposal of a broken bulb and you'll realize you need a Hazmat suit every time you change one or throw it away. Purchasing CFL bulbs to help conserve energy and save the environment doesn't make a lot of sense if we're polluting our earth with hazardous waste in order to do it.

Regular incandescent light bulbs are much healthier and safer, which makes them the lighting of choice in our house, at least for now. But keep an eye on the future of home lighting—it might be LED, which has energy-saving properties without the toxins. Of course, the cheapest light source of all—at least during the day—is to open those blinds and let the sun shine in.

> Read the instructions on a CFL box about the disposal of a broken bulb and you'll realize you need a Hazmat suit every time you change one or throw it away.

The Unnatural Need for Clean

Before the 1900s most of the dirt that made its way into homes was good old-fashioned mud, leaves, manure, and other organic material tracked in from the barnyard or street. A broom, a mop, and bucket of soapy water would pretty much do the trick for a thorough cleaning. Today, however, much of our "dirt" is made up of toxic residues that come from our synthetic "cleaning" solutions.

{ The germs in our homes are *our* germs. Our bodies generally have no problem dealing with the familiar. }

We've become obsessed with living in a germ-free environment as a result of the scare tactics employed by marketers. We have a bona fide germ phobia when we could be focusing our energy on something positive, like boosting our immune systems.

Let's put some things into perspective. Your body, when healthy, is beautifully designed to handle germs. The germs in our homes are *our* germs. Our bodies generally have no problem dealing with the familiar. We don't need to live in a scrubbed-down, sterilized bubble.

It's inconvenient to catch a cold, but we need to consider what having a common cold means in comparison to developing chronic degenerative diseases, which can result from the overuse of antibacterial cleaners. When you compare the discomfort of a sore throat to the risk of developing cancer, heart disease, or stroke, don't you think it's time for a new paradigm shift?

"Use the blue stuff on the glass, the purple stuff on the sink, the green stuff on the dishes and the ..."

We use sterilizing agents in the hope of avoiding a cold or flu, but those agents don't go away in just a few days. Solvents that break down organic matter will also break down the same sorts of molecules you find on your skin and in your lungs. They *need to* be toxic in order to kill the germs.

And yet you put yourself in contact with that stuff, touching and breathing it in the name of health.

We should never have to suck down toxic fumes just to be convinced that the cleaners we're using are effective. When you are using chemicals that you know produce dangerous substances, you should always take special precautions. Just because you are in the "safety" of your own home doesn't mean that these hazards can be taken lightly. In 2008, 214,230 human exposures to household cleaning products were reported to poison control centers in the United States, with another 100,000-plus exposures to pets.[2] Those who spend the most time in the home—the very young and the old as well as pregnant women—are most susceptible to poisoning from household cleaners.

You are not likely to find much information on the health hazards from indoor air in the home because the studies haven't been done, even though millions and millions have been spent investigating "sick building syndrome" when it's an office setting or industrial site. Once again, the most vulnerable—and most precious—are left behind.

Marketing is powerful. Advertisers once convinced us that smoking cigarettes had calming benefits and that chewing tobacco was a great smokeless alternative. With the right amount of money and enough loveable cartoon characters or celebrities to act as spokespeople, anything will sell. We all know it, yet we're still gullible. We *want to believe* because, quite frankly, cleaning is a pain—it feels as if we're being punished, and it takes away from our time to play.

We're always hopeful that a new product is going to make housekeeping chores less time consuming and less annoying.

Why would we think the windows won't be streak-free unless the spray has blue dye in it? Yet, if we really stop to think about it, wouldn't a clear liquid make a much better glass cleaner than the one with blue dye? Clear white vinegar is a perfectly effective window cleaner, one that's been used since the time glass was invented.

For centuries, humans around the globe have kept their homes sanitary without the beloved blue solution or powerful purple product. But today we think that stronger is always better. I have an employee who admits that she's always loved scrubbing a bathroom until her eyes water. If your nose burns, the room must be really clean, right?

Wrong.

Use your keenest sense of danger—your nose. Your body is yelling "Step away! Now!" We've learned to ignore these natural warning signals because we want a bathroom that smells clean or, in other words, smells like chemicals.

Your best tools for healthy cleaning

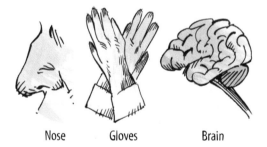

Nose   Gloves   Brain

This brings us back to the question of what it is that we are hoping to accomplish. At its most basic level, the goal of scrubbing is to maintain a healthy environment with a one-two-punch approach:

Ask the Scientist

"Dr. Wentz, why are children more susceptible to toxins?"

Several factors make children more vulnerable to toxic substances in air, water, food, and other sources as well as expose them to more toxins than adults must contend with each day.

From infancy onward, children eat more food, drink more fluids, and breathe more air than adults. Pound for pound, a baby girl under twelve months of age will consume twice as much food as a seven to twelve-year-old girl, and four times what a young woman over nineteen will eat. Children also breathe more rapidly and take in a relatively larger volume of air per minute than adults. Not only do they have a higher baseline rate of breathing, children breathe rapidly more often, especially during play.

Children are just setting out on the journey of life. They are constantly exploring their world through hearing and vision, as adults usually do, but also through taste, smell, and touch. The younger they are, the more time they spend on the floor or on the ground, where toxins tend to settle and accumulate.

It has long been known that organs and tissues that are still developing are more sensitive to damage from toxic influences. The immature gastrointestinal tract and blood-brain barrier in children allow

1) Remove toxins
2) Eliminate an environment favorable to molds, fungi, and bacteria

Chemical solutions happen to be the antithesis of both by adding toxins and encouraging the rampant spread of resistant superbugs.

Clean Contact

In addition to the terrible fumes, you also have to worry about coming into physical contact with the cleaner. When you clean with bleach or ammonia, you think it's all gone as soon as your nose becomes desensitized to the fumes.

for greater absorption of toxics. And their yet-undeveloped hepatic and renal functions are less efficient at metabolizing and excreting toxins. Children also have less protection due to their immature immune systems.

Children have a longer remaining lifetime to accumulate today's increased toxics, and they are developing degenerative diseases earlier in life. Increased exposure to toxins, combined with their heightened vulnerability, form the basis for my prediction years ago that children today will have a shorter life expectancy than their parents.

Yet we—and our children especially—constantly come into contact with surfaces all around the house. My son Andrew touches, bites, or sucks on *everything*. He is coming into contact with almost every surface of the house, and he is the one who's the most susceptible to toxins, given his hyper-speed growth and development.

There are many, many chemicals in ordinary household cleaners that are seriously dangerous, but no one knows exactly *how* dangerous because there are 80,000 chemicals registered with the EPA—far too many to be tested for safety. And we didn't want to slow innovation with cumbersome safety testing. Once again, the government chooses economy over ecology.

The same concept we discussed for beauty products applies to cleaning products—the effects are cumulative. Toxins build up in our bodies over time until we need a new term like "body burden." We simply don't have time to wait for science to produce data alerting us to the effects of this chronic, low-dose, lifetime exposure. We need to take action now.

Let's start with a quick inventory of the cleaners in your home. Check all the cleaners you currently use or often purchase.

- ❑ All-purpose cleaners
- ❑ Automatic dishwashing detergents
- ❑ Carpet cleaners
- ❑ Carpet fresheners
- ❑ Granite cleaners
- ❑ Stovetop scrubs
- ❑ Stainless steel sprays/wipes
- ❑ Chlorine bleach
- ❑ Degreasers
- ❑ Furniture polishes
- ❑ Dishwashing liquids
- ❑ Disinfecting wipes
- ❑ Drain clog removers
- ❑ Window cleaners
- ❑ Mold and mildew removers
- ❑ Oven cleaners
- ❑ Scouring cleansers

It's a little surprising to see just how many cleaning products you really use,

If you are a pet owner, you should be aware that animals are similarly affected by the toxic chemicals in cleaning products. Learn more at www.myhealthyhome.com/pets.

Cellular Truths

The Dangers of Mixing Household Cleaners

Mixing household cleaners—especially ammonia (often found in glass cleaners) with bleach—can produce a deadly cocktail. Bleach is a 5 percent solution of sodium hypochlorite ($NaOCl$). If this is mixed with ammonia (NH_3), chloramines are formed (NH_2Cl and NH_2Cl_2). In water these will further decompose to ammonia gas and hypochlorous acid.

The gases of chloramines, chlorine, and ammonia are extremely volatile, corrosive substances. In your airways, they will cause your lung cells to dissolve and your lungs to fill with fluid. Death can follow quickly if you do not vacate the area you are cleaning immediately.

Bleach mixed with a phosphate cleaner will release chlorine gas—also known as mustard gas—as well as hypochlorous acid. Hypochlorous acid reacts with a wide variety of biomolecules, including DNA, RNA, fatty acids, cholesterol, and proteins.

Sodium hypochlorite and organic chemicals—for example, surfactants and fragrances—common to most household cleaning products, can react with ammonia to generate chlorinated VOCs. Levels of chloroform and carbon tetrachloride in household air

right? That's why we recommend that you cut them *by at least half*.

Warning labels rarely show skulls and crossbones these days, but they will still quietly say, "Harmful if swallowed."

increase significantly whenever bleach is used. Both of these chemicals are recognized carcinogens and highly hazardous toxicants that affect neurological, cardiovascular, and respiratory systems.

Simple Solution:
If you are cleaning with products that you wouldn't eat, wear gloves!

However, even if you don't taste the tile scrub or guzzle the blue stuff, particles of cleaning solutions are still entering your bloodstream as they are absorbed through the skin on your hands as you scrub, on your feet as you walk across the floor, and on the rest of your body while you soak in the tub.

If you are having second thoughts about clean versus healthy, keep in mind that most chemicals in use today have been created in the last seventy-five years. You should clean with ingredients that have been used for hundreds of years and have shown no known toxic effects.

The Real Smell of Clean

Not only do we think things are getting cleaner if we smell harsh bleach and ammonia fumes, we also tend to believe that if we can't smell anything, there's nothing really there. And just as we use sticky dryer sheets to make our clothes smell fresh and clean, we also use carpet deodorizers and air fresheners to mask foul odors.

Simple Solution:
Instead of using an aerosol freshening spray, mist your room with real citrus scent. Simply pour a few drops of orange, lemon, or lime essential oil into a spray bottle of water.

Yet the bad odors are still there. We've just covered them with chemicals that are more powerful and smell more appealing. Both the odors and the chemicals are being sucked into our lungs, though, from which they get distributed throughout the body.

Greener Cleaners

In this book, the products we encourage you to clean with are nontoxic and biodegradable, which generally means they are plant based. Detergents should also be free of phosphates, which often end up in our freshwater lakes and cause algae blooms that rob the water of oxygen and kill wildlife. Virtually all laundry detergents are phosphate-free, but phosphates are still found in many dishwashing detergents.

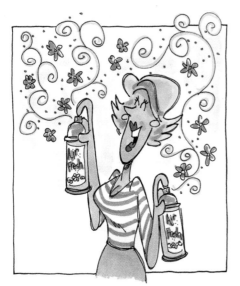

"Ahh, smells just like naphthalene, phenol, and pinene, with a touch of formaldehyde."

It's hard to go *au naturale* in our homes because we're so obsessed with all those germs. How can plain soap and vinegar rival the germ-killing powers of a harsh disinfectant? Traditional cleaners work well because they embody many of the fundamental aspects of the world itself—especially the nature of dirt.

The following cleaning solutions may not have the millions of dollars of marketing behind them, and they don't come in bright colors, but they do have generations of proof behind them.

Water

The universal solvent, water will get rid of most stains with a little effort and determination, but with no leftover residue.

Natural soaps

Castile soaps made from plant oils are mild but versatile cleaners, providing natural degreasing power.

Natural acidic solutions

Lemon juice is an example of a natural acidic cleaner. If you have an alkaline residue such as rust, soap scum, or water spots, the first approach to cleaning would be with an acidic solution, such as vinegar. (Do not use acidic cleaners on stone.)

- *White distilled vinegar* is a mild acid that readily dissolves soap scum, cleans glass, disinfects surfaces, and is a perfect natural fabric softener. Use white vinegar because apple cider or wine vinegar can stain.
- *Lemon juice* is a mild acid that also has mild bleaching properties. It is a great stain remover and whitener. Fresh squeezed lemon juice is best, but bottled lemon juice can also be used.

Natural alkaline solutions

Baking soda, cornstarch, club soda, and salt are alkaline solutions that work well to clean acidic problems like body oil, food stains, and general dirt and grime.

- *Baking soda (sodium bicarbonate)* is nature's most versatile cleaning product, a natural substance that has been used around the world for nearly 150 years to remove odors, soften water, dissolve dirt and grime, scrub soap scum, and even unclog drains.[3]
- *Borax (sodium borate)* is a mineral similar in properties to baking soda, but it has a higher pH and is, therefore, stronger. It can remove odors, soften water, and dissolve dirt. In addition, it has antifungal and antibacterial properties and can stop the growth of mold and mildew. Although natural, borax can be used as an insecticide to eliminate cockroaches, fleas, and ants. Knowing this, we can surmise that it is toxic if ingested and must be kept out of the reach of children. You can find borax near the other laundry detergents.[4]

■ *Club soda* (with *sodium citrate*) is handy for loosening dirt and softening water so that it dries without water spots. This inexpensive fizzy water is great for cleaning glass and appliances and removing stains from fabrics.

Essential oils

These concentrated oils contain the aroma of the plants from which they are made. Some common essential oils include eucalyptus, tea tree, lavender, lemon, orange, and peppermint. When added with lemon oil and distilled water, eucalyptus oil is an effective antibacterial spray. Lavender and tea tree oils are not only pleasantly calming, they too have been shown to have antibacterial and antifungal properties. Lemon and orange oil are nature's deodorizers. Essential oils come in small bottles, but you use just a few drops at a time so the supplies last a long time. However, be careful to avoid having them directly touch the skin.[5]

Elbow grease

Otherwise known as good old-fashioned physical effort, it will work wonders. Don't fall for the television ads that proclaim cleaning instantly with no effort. Without the powerful—and toxic—ingredients in many commercial cleaners, you can expect to work a little harder. But your health (and the health of your family) will be worth it.

Finally, sunshine—the oldest cleaning agent of all

Take a shirt that you've worn for a few hours—making sure that it isn't soiled or stained—and hang it in the sun in a well-ventilated spot. The next morning you'll likely decide that it really does fit the description of "clean." And it's been deodorized and disinfected as well.

Some of the most basic items in your cleaning kit are either acid or alkaline, and you use the respective solution on stains or compounds that are the opposite: acid cleaning for alkaline residue, and vice versa. What you are doing essentially is neutralizing the thing you want to remove, bringing it closer to nonacid or nonalkaline.

And what is the neutral cleaning solution? Water, at pH 7.0. When you have neutralized a compound with an acid or alkaline, you can rinse it out or away with water.

After getting the lowdown on dirt and what ingredients you need to get rid of it, it's not a surprise to find many healthy cleaners that work as well as your name-brand toxins. Why buy a blue window cleaner that contains vinegar as an extra cleaning ingredient when vinegar alone will do the job? Don't buy commercial cleaners for the fragrance, either. Toxic residue is far too high a price for a moment of flowery blast. Instead, create an effective and nontoxic window cleaning solution by simply mixing water, lemon juice, and vinegar.

Most natural cleaners actually cost less than commercial products— after all, *somebody's* got to pay for all that advertising—and when you combine the cost to the environment with your out-of-pocket expense, you'll find that you're coming out far ahead when you use "green" cleaners instead of blue ones.

Simple Homemade Solutions

With just a few inexpensive ingredients you can find in almost any grocery store, you can clean your whole house. These are healthy versions of all those colorful cleaners you waste money on at the store. It's time to clean, not contaminate.

- *All-purpose cleaner:* One quart of warm water plus 4 tablespoons baking soda, plus 1 teaspoon vinegar.
- *Carpet stain remover:* Baking soda plus water or club soda.
- *Window cleaner:* Three cups water plus a quarter cup of white vinegar and 1½ tablespoons of lemon juice. This magic formula is the new magical blue, without the blue.
- *Wood polish:* Two parts vegetable or olive oil plus 1 part lemon juice. Must be refrigerated.
- *Drain cleaner:* Combine ½ cup baking soda and ½ cup white vinegar. Pour the mixture down the drain. Next, pour a pot of boiling water down the drain to dissolve blockages caused by food particles, soap, and grease.
- *Stainless steel polisher:* Use baking soda and a soft-sided sponge. Toothpaste works too. Hey, maybe you've found a new use for your fluoridated toothpaste.
- *Heavy duty cleaning (for large jobs):* Add 1 teaspoon baking soda and 2 teaspoons of liquid soap to 1 gallon of hot water. If it's particularly stubborn, add 1 or 2 tablespoons of borax.
- *Disinfectant spray (also works on mildew):* Combine 2 cups water, ¼ cup tea tree oil, ¼ cup lavender oil. Use as a spray and let dry.

For more cleaning recipes, go to
www.myhealthyhome.com/cleaners.

The Welcome Mat

It is almost comical how paranoid we are about sterilizing our kitchen counters and bathrooms, yet we walk around unwittingly in car oil, pesticides, animal waste, and cleaners and other toxins just before we come traipsing through the front door.

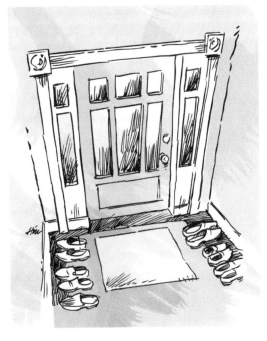

So at the Wentz house we leave a big pile of shoes at the front door as a signal to everyone that shoes and their collections of yuck aren't welcome in our home. My baby is going to be sitting on that floor my guests just walked across. His little hands are on the tile, wood, and carpet and then go straight into his mouth. Sure, the new germ exposure is helping him build his immune system, but I'd rather not introduce him to every germ out there all at once.

Let's face it: We don't have to be meticulous housekeepers to acknowledge that we drag a lot of strange stuff in on our shoes. So keep the shoes next to the door. Going barefoot will extend the life of your hardwood floors as well.

Get Steamed

Even if you're not tracking the world's mess into your home sweet home, you'll still want to clean your floors from time to time. One of the best devices you can use is a steam cleaner—also known as a vapor cleaner—which does its job without the use of toxic chemicals. This is definitely a worthwhile investment for eliminating dust mites and mold, which will help those people who suffer from allergies or multiple-chemical sensitivity.

Look for a vapor steam cleaner that produces "dry steam"—one that has a boiler temperature of at least 240° Fahrenheit.

Suck It Up

Is your vacuum cleaner healthy?

Household dust contains bacteria, mold spores, pollen grains, dust mites, and many other allergy triggers as well as many potentially toxic substances. Most vacuums release some of the dust they collect back into the air. Choose a brand that uses a true HEPA filter to trap microscopic particles and the majority of airborne allergens.

The best vacuums are ones that completely trap dust and dirt—including allergens and chemical residues—and prevent them from escaping back into your home.

> **Simple Solution:**
> Buy the best vacuum you can afford. Optimally, get one with a HEPA "completely sealed" system.

Be aware that vacuums are a powerful source of EMFs. Thus, the less time you spend vacuuming and the greater distance you put between your body and the vacuum motor the better.

A similar danger comes when people wear a vacuum or leaf blower on their backs. They are placing themselves in dangerously close proximity to unhealthy electrical fields. Once again, find a vacuum with a canister and hose that allows you to put a little more space between you and the motor so you can reduce your ongoing exposure to EMFs.

Get Tested

No, this doesn't mean going into the doctor and giving blood. This is a simple and inexpensive—but potentially life-saving—act of having your home tested.

Everyone should, at a minimum, have their house tested for mold, radon, and lead, which are potentially dangerous elements that can be hiding there. It's sad how many news stories we hear of a father working in his basement and later dying from black mold. Even your sleek granite countertops may be emitting radiation and radon gas. You need to know if these dangers are lurking in your home so you can take steps to protect your family.

Getting your home tested for contaminants is easy and fairly inexpensive—*extremely* inexpensive compared to the medical bills you may avoid paying. You can go to your local home store and buy kits that will enable you to check for mold, radon, carbon monoxide, lead, and other toxins, or you can go online and find a professional service that will come out and test your home with methods ranging from mold-sniffing dogs to infrared equipment.

Chapter 11
High Tech, High Risk

During the past twenty-five years, we've witnessed incredibly rapid advancements in technology for the home, many of which have made our lives unbelievably convenient.

Worried about missing the big game? Hop on your mobile phone and send a signal to your DVR to record it. You don't have to worry about watching commercials either.

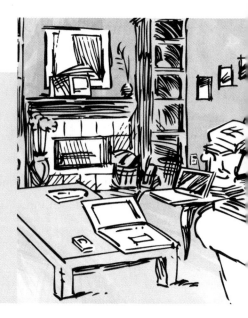

QUIZ

How Toxic Is Your Home?

Scores

1. What are the **two** most common methods you use for talking on the phone?
   - ☐ Corded landline (0 pts)
   - ☐ Landline on speaker (0 pts)
   - ☐ Cordless phone (2 pts)
   - ☐ Mobile phone (10 pts)
   - ☐ Mobile phone with Bluetooth® headset (6 pts)
   - ☐ Mobile phone with wired headset (3 pts)
   - ☐ Mobile phone using speaker (3 pts)

2. Imagine that you have been separated from your mobile phone for the day. (Let's say you left it at home or it has lost its charge.) How would you feel for those 10 hours?

   More relaxed than usual   ←————————————→   A nervous wreck

   0 pts   8 pts   16 pts

3. How often do you get your heart rate up from physical activity? (Select one)
   - ☐ Daily (0 pts)
   - ☐ A few times a week (2 pts)
   - ☐ Weekly (5 pts)
   - ☐ A few times a month (8 pts)
   - ☐ Never (12 pts)

4. Have you switched your home's lighting to compact fluorescent bulbs?

   All   Half   None

   10 pts   5 pts   0 pts

Your "High Tech" danger score:

1–12	13–24	25–36	37+
The brightest bulb	Low-wattage	Fizzling fast	Burned out

Need to make a flight reservation? Access the Internet from your laptop while lying in bed and send your boarding pass to your wireless printer.

Feel bored or lonely? Power up a video game and you can compete for hours with a stranger halfway around the world.

Worried about a looming deadline? Connect with your office computer from home and re-immerse yourself in the project you just left at work. It's all so incredibly easy! Yet with each leap in technology and its apparent benefits, we face unintended consequences in our physical and emotional health.

Gadgets Galore

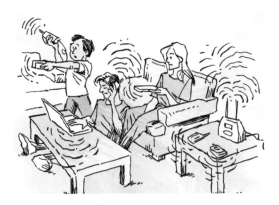

As an admitted gadget geek, I constantly have to temper my enthusiasm for the latest technological breakthrough with my knowledge that there are downsides to progress. Some of the devices that make our life easier are also making us fat, depressed, alienated, and sick. That's not to say that we should go back to horses and buggies, the eight-track, the Walkman, or even dial-up Internet. Change is the only thing we can really count on in life, but that shouldn't stop us from examining the potentially negative effects and minimizing any risks. We owe it to ourselves—and especially our children—to find a happy medium between progress and safety, tech time and family time, the virtual world and the natural world, and work and play.

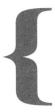
Some of the devices that make our lives easier are also making us sick, fat, depressed, and alienated.

In many ways, technology has become the enemy to intimacy. We regularly text our spouses, mealtimes at home have become pit stops, we have TVs and laptops in the bedroom, and there's less face-to-face interaction between us and our families, friends, and even strangers.

Recently Reneé and I were sitting at a mall and watching what looked like an impending collision. A college-aged man and woman walked straight toward each other, both peering down at their phones, completely engrossed in texting. To Reneé it seemed like a scene straight out of a romantic comedy. Maybe their fates had aligned to bring the two of them together. After smacking right into each other, they'd laugh out their apologies, introduce themselves, flirt a little, and live happily ever after.

But at the very last second, without looking up or acknowledging each other, they nimbly stepped to the side and kept right on texting. Though we were impressed with the last-minute maneuvering, we also wondered if they'd missed out on a real connection.

Our gadgets aren't just robbing us of human connections, though. They also might be posing a *physical* threat to our health and longevity.

A Sea of Radiation

Every living space in our homes is filled with technological instrumentation that place us at risk. In chapter 2, we covered the health dangers associated

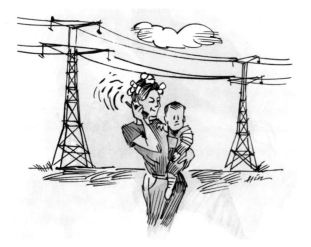

with electromagnetic fields (EMFs) created by electronics such as lamps, alarm clocks, and electric blankets. But there's a steadily growing risk from an even higher source of EMF exposure—radio frequency (RF) emissions.

As mentioned in the bedroom section, RF fields are created by some of our most modern conveniences, including mobile phones and Wi-Fi. The increase in the use of these electronic gadgets continues at full speed. In fact, as this book is being written, there are an estimated four billion cell phone users around the globe, and as many as a third of them are children. Both numbers are certain to grow.

Mobile phone users are exposed to intense levels of RF radiation that are significantly higher than those found naturally in the environment. A cellular phone is basically a radio that sends RF signals to a distant base station—as well as to your central nervous system. It easily penetrates the tissues of the brain and other organs. Other wireless communication devices such as Wi-Fi are similar, as these devices also radiate microwave signals.[1]

{ A cellular phone is basically a radio that sends RF signals to a distant base station—as well as to your central nervous system. }

Scientists postulate that the human body responds to these energy fields as invading pathogens, setting in place a cascade of biochemical reactions that cause the release of damaging free radicals, alter the blood-brain barrier, kick-start chronic inflammatory responses, and disrupt intercellular communications.

The U.S. National Toxicology Program notes that current exposure guidelines are limited to protection from thermal injuries—in essence, the radio waves actually heating or burning your skin—but concedes that evidence of other adverse effects is now emerging.[2] The agency is conducting studies focusing on possible cancer-causing or other toxic effects. The Interphone Project, an international series of epidemiological studies conducted by thirteen participating countries, has begun to release interim results. And some studies associate certain cancers of the head—acoustic neuroma and glioma—with prolonged cell phone use.[3]

As stated in chapter 2, almost twenty years after cellular communication was introduced to the global market, we are reaching the end of the latency period for cancers to appear, and the scientific evidence is quickly mounting that cell phone use *is* associated with the development of serious adverse health effects.

Mini-mobilers

With concern growing over the risks of using mobile phones, we can't help but worry about our kids. Most children use their thumbs to text message faster than adults can type on conventional keyboards. It's not uncommon to see kids "chatting" away, well before they've entered the teenage years. There is no denying that for teens and tweens, a hand-held, wireless world is here.

As the use of these devices grows, so does the evidence that the electromagnetic fields they emit present much greater hazards than previously thought, especially for those whose bodies and brains are still developing. Dr. Lennart Hardell, a cancer expert from University Hospital in Sweden, recently found that among individuals who began using cell phones before they were twenty years old, after a year or more of use, the risk of brain cancer was 5.2 times greater than for the general population.[4]

Though the most common concern is cancer, there are other serious hazards. A 2008 study from the UCLA School of Public Health asked more than 13,000 mothers to complete a questionnaire that included questions about the health and behavioral status of their children at seven years of age. It also asked whether the mothers had used cell phones during the pregnancy or immediately after the birth. By nearly two-to-one, the children whose mothers reported cell phone use during this critical time demonstrated behavioral difficulties such as hyperactivity around the age they entered school.[5]

It took seventy years to remove lead from paint and gasoline, and fifty years to establish the link between smoking and cancer and to have warnings printed on packs of cigarettes. Even the ancient Greeks noted that asbestos was harmful, but it took the United States more than sixty years to ban its use after illnesses were documented.

Isn't it about time for us to learn our lesson and see if we can avoid a pandemic of brain tumors?

When it comes to protecting our most valuable heritage, it's time to employ the precautionary principle we discussed in section 1. You can either conclude cell phones are safe until proven dangerous, or you can call on your intuition where as many as a billion children and young adults are involved and take a few simple precautions that could make a huge difference.

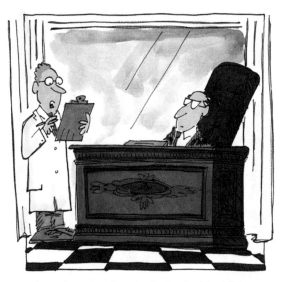

"Your three-month study of 1,000 healthy children using cell phones proved conclusively that they are completely safe with zero cases of cancer created."

Andrew loves our cell phones, and we don't mind letting him play with them when they are in "airplane mode." We don't want the transmission scrambling the cockpit (his brain). Otherwise, we don't plan to allow him to use a cell phone while he's young, *except* in the case of emergencies. Parents must remember that the brains of infants and small children aren't protected by the same fully developed skulls that we have.

Learn which wireless devices have the lowest emissions at www.myhealthyhome.com/wireless.

And kids will be subjected to many more years of cell phone exposure than we were.

Let's do what we can to minimize their exposure in their earliest years.

Protecting Yourself and Your Family

It's become difficult to see how we can manage without cell phones and other wireless technologies—I love my iPhone just as much as the next person. However, it pays to use common sense. As with all forms of EMFs, the farther away you are from the source of RF radiation, the lower your level of exposure will be.

Simple Solution:

If your child just can't resist playing with your mobile phone, turn it off first. Or if you have a smartphone, you can switch it to "airplane mode."

My father has long suspected the dangers posed by wireless and cordless phones and generally refuses to hold them next to his head. He prefers to talk on a speaker phone, which can be a bit disconcerting if you're trying to have a private conversation. However, speaker phone quality has come a long way in recent years, and we could all stand to use it more often.

I personally try to spend as little time talking on the cell phone as possible. I'll ask people to call back using the landline, or I'll send a text so I don't have

Ask the Scientist

"Dr. Wentz, are there negative health effects caused by radio frequencies coming from cell phones?"

On the subject of electromagnetic radiation, the one thing there's no shortage of is opinions.

When you consider the pervasiveness of cell phone users around the world, it should be no surprise that there are plenty of arguments on both sides of the debate. But there are some facts that can't be denied by either side.

First, each and every day we are exposed to radiation levels many times higher than existed just a generation ago. We are surrounded by cell phones, wireless Internet, cordless phones, garage door openers, baby monitors, laptop computers, microwave ovens, and even fluorescent lighting.

Second, the current regulations addressing the health effects of electromagnetic radiation exposure are based on the conviction that only thermal effects are hazardous. We now know that to be wrong.

We know that some forms of radiation—such as x-rays—are undeniably lethal. What about other forms, such as the RF radiation emitted by cell phones? It is only a billionth of the intensity of x-rays, but it's stronger than FM radio signals. Is the poison in the

to hold the phone up to my head.

Many of us keep our phones in a belt clip or in a pocket, exposing our hip bones and major organs to radiation. If RF fields are indeed messing with our blood's DNA, this could be doing a lot of damage to our long-term health. One simple way to address this is to constantly alternate where you carry your cell phone, to spread the exposure around and not concentrate it day-in and day-out in one crucial spot. Women who carry purses already put some distance between themselves and their phones. If you don't carry a purse, look for other ways to maintain your distance. Keep your cell phone on your desk or on your dashboard—just not in your pocket.

Another easy way to minimize overall exposure is to use a wired, hands-free headset for your phone and keep the phone at least a couple feet away from your head and any other body parts, including your lap. The *wired* part is important, because wireless headsets act as miniature wireless transmitters, so by using them you're not doing as much to protect your brain.

dose, or do we need to take into consideration the fact that x-ray exposure lasts only an instant, whereas we are subjected to RFs of some sort virtually every moment in our lives?

The question of the health effects of RF radiation simply can't be answered accurately yet. It's like a jigsaw puzzle, and we still haven't been given all the pieces. The evidence of potential damage is growing, but hard, scientific answers aren't likely to be available for years.

Should we wait that long?

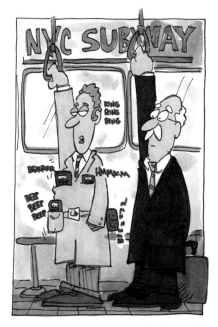

"No, I'm not a stock broker. I'm a waiter."

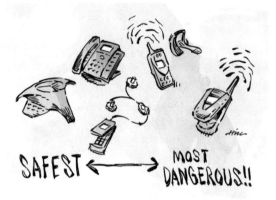

SAFEST ←——→ MOST DANGEROUS!!

And though many people wonder if they should even bother with a landline at home anymore, I encourage you to keep it and—most importantly—use it.

The greatest concern, however, is our obsession with never being out of touch. We take our phones *everywhere*, and people almost tremble with fear when they have to turn off their phones. Teenagers sleep with the phone under the pillow so they won't miss a late night call or text. Many people keep it on their nightstand so they can respond immediately if it vibrates or blinks.

> **Simple Solution:**
> Use a regular, corded telephone when at home or at work. Cutting even 20 percent of your daily RF exposure is a step in the right direction.

Why Wi-Fi?

Wi-Fi is increasingly difficult to get away from these days. It's on planes, in coffee shops and restaurants, and in most workspaces and hotel rooms. But you can choose to eliminate it from the one place you can control—your home.

If you really, really need the convenience of Wi-Fi, just consider turning it off so it's not transmitting when you don't need it. Use that "off" switch or pull the plug. Most people don't need Wi-Fi for the third of their life that they are sleeping.

I'll confess that I'm one of those people who opted for Wi-Fi. It's convenient, though, especially in a home that's a converted warehouse with few interior walls and limited wiring. I've made a conscious decision in favor of the convenience of working on my

> **Simple Solution:**
> If you have Ethernet ports in convenient areas, you can access the Internet using good, old-fashioned wiring.

laptop anywhere in the home, despite the risk of exposing myself to more RF emissions. However, I've also opted to store all the major electronics—including the Wi-Fi box—in one spot that's on the opposite side of our home from the bedroom, the nursery, and the kitchen. And we're keeping our son as far away from this high-tech hotspot during the time his brain and body are still developing.

It's interesting that we call public Wi-Fi areas "hotspots." We should hope that term isn't given more meaning in the future if they find it to be dangerous like a nuclear "hotspot."

The Great Electronic Depression

Not all of the modern world's dangers are physical.

Although not yet accepted as a defined disease, excessive online activity has been labeled as "Internet addiction." With one billion personal computers in use worldwide as of 2008, and another billion expected to be in use by 2015,[6] the issue of Internet addiction is almost certain to become more problematic. The constant need to be online—and its negative health effects—serve as frightening warnings about the ugly trade-offs we often make in order to enjoy technological advancement.

Internet Addiction

Internet addiction is basically pathological computer dependency with at least three distinct variants—gambling, pornography, and excessive e-mailing/text messaging. We will lump social media usage into this last area.[7]

Regardless of the online activity, people with Internet addiction usually exhibit the following "symptoms":

- Excessive use, frequently punctuated by a loss of the sense of time and a neglect of basic physical needs such as eating, sleeping, bathing, and physical activity
- Withdrawal, including symptoms such as anger, depression, and anxiety when the computer cannot be accessed

- Increasing tolerance, basically amounting to an obsession with obtaining more and better computer equipment and software, or more hours of computer use
- Negative repercussions, such as social isolation, lack of interest in other endeavors, and poor performance at work or school[8]

Few large-scale epidemiological studies examining problematic Internet use—in essence, Internet usage that goes beyond the healthy norm—have been completed. However, existing data suggest that Internet addiction is a global phenomenon, impacting people of nearly all age groups in numbers approaching those of schizophrenia and bipolar disorder.[9]

Simple Solution:
Keep an "open door" policy when it comes to online activity for children or teens. In other words, no surfing behind locked doors.

Yet computers and the Internet are an integral part of life for kids today. And teenagers are extremely vulnerable to addictive disorders, based on social *and* neurobiological factors. For this reason, you must remain vigilant for signs of problematic computer use in the adolescents and young adults in your life.

> People aren't spending as much time in their "real lives" with family, friends, and school or professional obligations. A preoccupation with the Internet can lead to depression and feelings of isolation.

All of this virtual interaction means that people aren't spending as much time in their "real lives" with family, friends, and school or professional obligations. A preoccupation with the Internet can lead to depression and feelings of isolation, and the social consequences, like academic failures, job losses, financial difficulties, legal problems, family conflicts, and divorce, can send a person even further into online seclusion.[10]

You can help offset this issue in your own home by limiting technology time—especially for children—and addressing as early as possible any computer usage that feels like it could become a problem. And remember that you set the example for your children and grandchildren. If you never truly disengage from your computers and Blackberrys, how can you expect your kids to do so?

Although most of us don't struggle with a true Internet addiction, we should honestly and frequently assess the impact that technology is having on our health and relationships. Start by asking yourself the following questions:

- How often do you let the distractions of the Web eat up hours of your day?
- What or who are you ignoring when you're online?
- Can you enjoy an evening at home without logging on or constantly checking that Blackberry or iPhone?
- Do you often miss out on fun moments with family or skip healthy outdoor activities in order to be on Facebook or Twitter?
- Do you regularly suffer from physical soreness or stiffness because of your technology time?

If technology is getting in the way of your job, family life, or health, it might be time to get help from a counselor.

Simple Solution:
Try to confine business to specific hours and areas, and consider setting aside a block of time each day in which you're technology-free and instead plugged-in to the real world.

Simple Solutions Summary

As Reneé and I slowly weaned ourselves from lemon-scented dust spray and sinus-clearing toilet bowl cleaner over the past few years, we've both noticed something interesting: Those cleaning products that once smelled so great are now almost nauseating with their cloying perfumes and eye-watering ingredients. Our noses are now telling us the toxic truth.

Although we now pride ourselves on our green-cleaned home, it wasn't necessarily an easy switch. Like most worthwhile science projects, the Great Cleaning Experiment (as I like to refer to it) featured many frustrating failures. There was the summer of static—in which our laundered clothes seemed to create EMFs of their very own. And there were several rounds of bizarrely sticky floors as we searched for just the right recipe for mopping our home's tile.

But when we watched Andrew make his first successful crawl across that same floor, we knew our hard work was worth it.

Our cleaning habits aren't the only thing to change. The fact that I was even home that evening to see Andrew make his first successful attempt at crawling is a testament to my efforts to set technological boundaries for myself. As a CEO, I know how difficult it is to get away from the office. Technology has made it so our jobs are always with us. It took years for me to learn that an e-mail, text message, or phone call could wait until morning. I used to get out of bed when I heard the ding of a new e-mail popping into my inbox. But I've realized that I'm not a doctor on call, and work can wait until morning. We all need to know the difference between being available to our coworkers and working the 411 information shift, 24/7.

Still, I look forward to the rare times when I am completely unplugged. I have been fortunate enough to travel all over the world and stay in some truly luxurious places. But when I'm asked about my favorite vacation spot, I don't hesitate: Lake Powell in southern Utah's beautiful red-rock country. I like to wakeboard and I love the scenery, but the real allure is the utter remoteness of the place. No mobile phone service, no Internet, no e-mails, no breaking news to interrupt fun and important moments with my family and friends. All of us should make a conscious decision, every so often, to disconnect from our gadgets and just *be* with the people we love. Real life's too incredible to let it slip by.

What Simple Solutions will you add to your Living Areas?

Scores

1. I will: (Select all that apply)
- Reduce current chemical cleaning products by at least half (8 pts)
- Wear rubber gloves every time when using cleaning products (5 pts)
- Switch to some of the natural homemade cleaners found in this book or online (5 pts)
- Eliminate the use of room/carpet fresheners (6 pts)

2. I will: (Select all that apply)
- Use a vacuum with a fully sealed HEPA filter system (10 pts)
- Get my home professionally tested for contaminants like radon, mold, carbon monoxide, and lead (10 pts)
- Switch from chemical hard-surface cleaners to a steam cleaner— one that uses only heated water (10 pts)

3. I will:
- Make all living areas a "no-shoe" zone and stick to it (10 pts)

4. I will: (Select all that apply)
- Stop all use of compact fluorescent bulbs (10 pts)
- If keeping compact fluorescent bulbs, I will learn (and use) proper disposal procedures in the case of a broken bulb (4 pts)

5. I will: (Select all that apply)
- Use the mobile speakerphone setting whenever possible (5 pts)
- Use a hands-free, wired headset with my mobile device (5 pts)
- Always use a landline from a corded telephone for calls from home and work (5 pts)
- Stop clipping the mobile phone to my belt or waistband (3 pts)
- Maintain a mobile-free rule—at least when the phone is transmitting— for kids under fourteen (10 pts)

6. I will: (Select all that apply)
- Use wired Internet at home instead of wireless (10 pts)
- Place the Wi-Fi router far from bedrooms and main living areas (3 pts)
- Shut off the Wi-Fi router at bedtime (5 pts)
- Set a "disconnect" time each day, when I shut off the computer, TV, and mobile phones (8 pts)

Your Simple Solutions positive score:

Your "Clean" danger score: -

Your "High Tech" danger score: -

Your Living Areas Health total:

You can track your quiz scores and solution points on *The Healthy Home* Web site at www.myhealthyhome.com.

Are you making a positive difference?

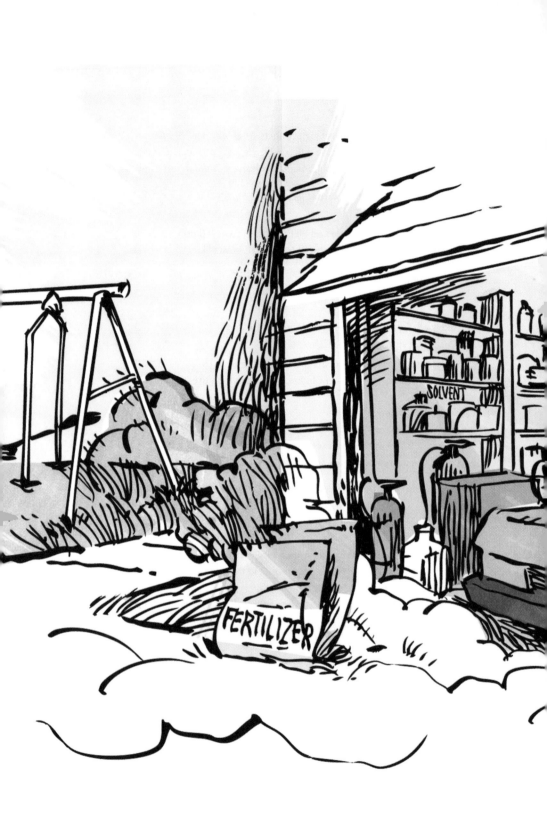

6

The Garage and Yard

Two areas just steps away from the walls of our homes can be real mine fields when it comes to major health concerns: the garage and the yard. The contaminants found in the garage, patio, yard, and beyond most assuredly influence life on the inside as well.

You may not feel as if you're ready to take on the whole world, but with a few simple changes, you can have a dramatic effect on your home's perimeter, establishing a barrier against the toxic substances that could make you and your family ill.

Even more rewarding, you can create an outdoor space that promotes relaxation, renewal, and wellness.

Our last stop takes us back out to where Dave's home meets the world beyond. Dave slides back a glass door and a screen, and we walk out onto a second-story patio that feels as large as the home we've just left. The private rooftop garden is reminiscent of an English courtyard. Birds chirp from mature trees that line the entire space, providing privacy and shade. Symmetric stone pathways cut through lush grass. Just down the street, a church bell begins to chime.

As we step outside, Dr. Wentz pulls another device out of his bag of tricks.

Donna: This makes your home truly unique. It's like having your very own park.

Dave: Thank you. Yes, this is what sold me on it. To live in the middle of city, within walking distance of everything, and yet still be able to grow tomatoes and play in the grass—it's the best.

Dr. Wentz: *[Holding up a small device that looks like a cable television remote control.]* And look at this VOC meter. Inside it was showing a low 0.4 parts per million reading, and when we come outside, though we're right downtown, the air is even cleaner at 0.2 parts per million.

Dave: Yep, one of my favorite additions in the whole remodel were these pull screens in the doors that let fresh air in but stop the insects that would tempt Reneé to get out the bug spray.

[Walking to the roof's edge, we look down at the passing cars.]

Donna: There doesn't seem to be a lot of parking available on the street. Do you have a garage around here?

Dave: We have a couple of private parking spaces nearby in the parking lot, but no garage.

Dr. Wentz: I've always told Dave that not having a garage is one of the best things about this place—at least when it comes to his family's health. My garage has caused me a fair number of headaches, I assure you.

Donna: Literally?

Dr. Wentz: Probably, but mainly it's been headaches that come from having to create safety measures. An attached garage is essentially another room in the house, and all the pollutants stored there escape to the rest of the house through gaps in the walls as well as anytime the connecting door is open. It's the equivalent of storing a car, automotive fluids, pesticides, fertilizers, and other garbage in an extra bedroom.

Dave: Despite all that, I wish for a garage every February when the snow really starts to come down. It would be nice in the middle of the summer, too.

Donna: Because your car gets so hot?

Dave: Exactly. Remember, heat accelerates the breakdown of plastic and other toxic materials. After baking in the sun, the interior of a car can release some pretty potent fumes; it's basically that "new car smell" that people like so much.

Donna: But that's one of the things people love about buying a new car!

Dave: I felt the same way until we had Andrew. Now I hate the idea.

Chapter 12
Gremlins in the Garage

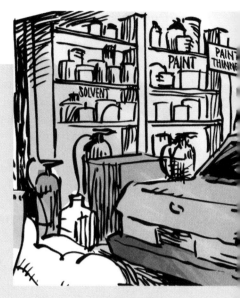

If there's one overriding concept about health we should all take away from this tour, it's to always be aware of the potential impact our immediate surroundings and activities can have on us. We should constantly be questioning what's in the food, water, air, and places where we live, work, and play.

This mindset shouldn't change when we step into the garage or walk out to the patio or yard.

QUIZ   How Toxic Is Your Home?   Scores

1. Do you have an attached garage? Yes_____ (8 pts)	
2. If you marked yes to question 1, please select all of the following that apply to your garage: ☐ The walls/ceiling are unfinished or just drywall (6 pts) ☐ Two or more vehicles pull in and out most days (6 pts) ☐ Small, gas-powered devices (lawnmower, snowblower, chain saw, etc.) are stored inside (2 pts each) ☐ Painting products and pesticides are stored there (5 pts)	
3. Select all of the following things that describe your vehicular habits. If you don't have a car, enter 0. ☐ Use the recirculated air button (3 pts) ☐ Use air fresheners of any kind (3 pts) ☐ Generally keep the windows rolled up (5 pts)	
4. If you selected one or more of the car habits on question 3, please select how much time you typically spend in your car each day: 30 minutes or less 1 hour 90 minutes 2 hours+ ◄——————┼————————┼————————► 0 pts 2 pts 4 pts 6 pts	
5. Do you or your spouse work on your own car? Yes_____ (6 pts)	

Your "Garage" danger score

1–10	11–20	21–30	31+
Zipping by	On cruise control	Check engine light	Stalled

Two-Car Bedroom

My dad and late night TV comedian Jay Leno have a common passion. They both have a love affair with automobiles, and both have unique garages.

Jay Leno's garage is a twenty-car museum and restoration facility. My father's garage, however, is more like a laboratory, organized and clean enough to double as a surgical suite, with every tool and gadget hung or stored according to function and accessibility. Every container has an airtight lid on it. Most importantly, he takes special care to ensure that neither the fumes from his cars nor chemicals or pollutants from

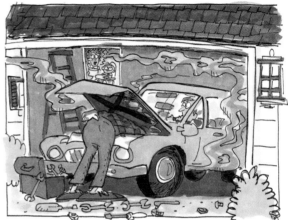

"Rev it up again for me, Johnny."

outside his home enter his living space. There was a time when I thought my dad was being extreme, but I've come to understand why he takes such precautions.

He's never grown accustomed to the garage being a part of the house.

His dad—my grandfather, Adam Wentz—was a farmer, but he was also a businessman. The family had a hardware store, a farm implement shop, and an auto dealership—places where my dad claims to have developed his love for high-performance vehicles and the hobby of browsing the garden section of hardware stores.

In America's past, our vehicles, workbenches, equipment, and chemicals were housed in "out-buildings," not to be confused with outhouses. On farms and ranches, all this stuff is still parked in barns, sheds, and garages, always some distance away from the family's home. As the national population expanded and the industrial revolution pushed the migration from rural areas to the cities, the cost of real estate increased and the size of residential lots decreased. Houses were built very close together, and the garages and storage areas were no longer kept in separate buildings.

When more people began living in cities, garages were predominantly found out back, just beyond the backyard, facing an alley. These small structures housed bicycles, greasy tools, trash cans, odds and ends, and dust-covered junk. If people were lucky, they were able to squeeze a car in as well.

Then came condos, townhouses, and suburbia. Not only did the number of pets and children begin decreasing, but so did the space that lay between garages and the main living space. For those of us in colder winter climates who have to scrape frost off the windshield or run through the rain with the groceries and kids, an attached garage seemed like a brilliant idea, especially for extra storage. Our tightly enclosed garages, often located just beneath the second-story bedrooms, likely contain two or more cars as well as the tool shop and a collection of old, crusty paint cans, thinners, cleaners, and glues we'll never use again.

Hold Your Breath

Attached garages are convenient and may even be a luxury, but there is growing evidence that they are responsible for adversely affecting the indoor air quality of our homes. The cars and products we store in our garages generate and leak substances that are considered toxic. Once these substances become airborne, they can easily migrate.

Car exhaust and other combustion pollutants, chemicals, and volatile organic compounds (VOCs) are present in most garages at least some of the time. And they can find their way into the house through open doors, gaps around closed doors, heating or cooling ducts, and other wall and ceiling connections. Numerous studies have found that homes with attached garages have higher levels of air pollutants—including benzene and carbon monoxide—than homes with no garage or a separate garage.[1]

Yet if you're like my dad and do have an attached garage, don't call the realtor or contractor just yet. There are some easy, do-it-yourself projects—along with some more complex solutions—that will help you breathe a whole lot easier.

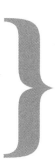

> Numerous studies have found that homes with attached garages have higher levels of air pollutants—including benzene and carbon monoxide—than homes with no garage or a separate garage.

Block It

To prevent contaminated air from passing into living spaces, make sure there's a good seal between garage and home. Start with the door that connects your garage to the rest of your living space. Apply weather stripping to ensure that it's sealed and closes tightly. Inexpensive self-closing hinges will help even the most harried parent—or forgetful child—keep the connecting door closed and garage toxins out of the home.

Next, seal the entire common wall as well as the ceiling between the garage and your home—including ductwork, wiring, and plumbing. Seal your ducts with water-based duct mastic compound and fill in the gaps around electrical work and wall-to-floor junctions with expanding spray foam and caulk.

Finish It

Don't assume that because your builder didn't finish the attached garage that it's not necessary to do so. Open walls and unfinished drywall are notoriously leaky. Make sure the walls *and* ceiling are hung with drywall, properly sealed, and given a couple coats of paint. You may have to contend with a few more VOCs from the paint, but in the long term you'll be providing much better protection against wandering garage fumes.

Clean It

Take a good look around your garage. Do you really need all of those products with "Warning," "Danger," and "Poison" on the label? When was the last time you actually used them? And given what you've learned, do you still feel good about employing them in your home?

Between the pesticides, paints, motor fluids, and heavy-duty cleaners sitting on shelves, many garages now resemble a chemical waste dump—but without the government oversight. Put on a good pair of gloves and maybe even a dust mask or respirator, and clean up.

Remember that most of these materials cannot be safely discarded at home. Call your local hazardous waste facility—or if you can't find one, look on your city or county government's Web site for sanitation or waste management services—to find out how and where to properly dispose of these dangerous materials. You'll know it's a government or nonprofit agency if they are ".gov" or ".org" Web sites and not ".com."

Cover It

You may need to keep a small can of paint around for touch-ups. But any potentially toxic items you keep should be properly sealed. Don't let cans of paint, paint thinner, solvents, gasoline, and other liquids sit around uncovered. And remember that once a container is opened, it's not possible to completely reseal it. A small amount of vapors will always escape into your garage, and then quite possibly into your living areas. If you've stored several opened cans there, then the accumulation of fumes could be dangerous.

Although not foolproof, a safer way to store paint is to place a layer of plastic wrap over the top of the paint can before replacing the lid. Tap down the lid with a rubber mallet, and then store the can of paint upside down. I recommend making any touch-up painting an annual task—for example, when you start your spring cleaning. That way you're not repeatedly opening the paint can and releasing fumes.

Air It

We all know not to leave the car running with the garage door closed, but idling isn't a safe practice even with the garage door open. Combustion pollutants are created and released every time you start a car, and if they make it into the house, you and your family will breathe them in.

For that reason, don't start your car until you're truly ready to get on the road, and then back out as immediately as you can. And when you return, shut the car off as soon as you pull into the garage. Your car will continue to emit some level of pollutants—more if the car is older—as the engine cools. All that exhaust in the garage has to go somewhere, but you can vent it outdoors by installing a fan or two. A basic bathroom or kitchen fan should do the trick, although there are more complex systems that start automatically when the garage door is opened and closed and stop on a timer system.

It's worth your time and money to install a fan, especially if you frequently work in your garage with wood finishes, paint, or other chemicals.

> **Simple Solution:**
> After a long drive, consider parking the car outside for an hour or two before moving it into the garage. Your engine will cool without polluting your garage and living areas.

Move It

Although most car engines today have a catalytic converter that helps reduce emissions, that's not the case with lawn mowers, outboard motors, snowblowers, and chain saws. Small, gas-powered devices can release serious amounts of gasoline-related pollutants, including the carcinogen benzene. In fact, walking behind your own roaring lawn mower can expose you to quite a lot of air pollution.

Small engines can emit pollutants even when they're not turned on. So if you have space for it, build a small shed away from the house for storing your portable, gasoline-powered equipment.

Toxic Hitchhikers

Toxins don't just waft in—they also *walk* in.

During my global travels as a business executive, especially in Asia, I've been impressed with the cultural practice of removing shoes before entering a home or apartment to avoid tracking in dirt and other contaminants. And when I return home after a week of airplane lavatories and dirty cabs, I'm reminded of why I remove my shoes each time I see Andrew smiling up at me from the kitchen floor.

Some houses have a "mudroom"—a small space you pass through before you enter the house itself. You can store your shoes there, and by keeping the mudroom easy to clean, you can avoid tracking anything in on your socks or bare feet.

For families who don't have a mudroom, the garage is a great place for a shoe rack or basket. As I mentioned in section 4, in my home we tend to just let shoes pile up in front of our front door, so guests get the picture without even being asked.

Eau du VOC

Thus far we've been focused on emissions from under a car's hood, but we also need to be aware of what emanates from a car's interior. It's a scent that signifies success, and we love to inhale it—that wonderful smell of newness we get when we can finally buy a brand new car.

But what is that smell and what creates it?

Unlike our laundry detergent, it's not from a chemist trying to fool us into believing we're smelling lavender and roses. Nope, this is the real deal. The scent of a new car is the off-gassing of fresh plastics, vinyls, leathers, paints, and synthetic carpets. And new car owners are

Ask the Scientist

"Dr. Wentz, are there any issues you deal with in your own garage?"

One important but often overlooked issue with a connected garage is the positioning of the garage relative to the house and prevailing winds in the area. The winds in our particular residential area come from the northwest. The problem is that the garage is on the north side of our home. So if I leave the garage door open and go into the house, the winds push the fumes right in with me.

Even with the doors closed, there is still movement.

I learned many years ago in my laboratories that protection is provided to living cells by controlling the air pressure in the room. You want positive air pressure in a clean room and negative pressure in a contaminated room. So it follows that your connected garage should be exhausted in such a way that you have negative pressure in the garage compared to the house. If you must gain entry to the house via the garage, you want the house air to be pulled into the garage rather than the dirty garage air pushed in your living space.

Keeping in mind that the garage has different fumes that are both heavier and lighter than air, the best way to vent an attached garage properly would be to have

sucking it down by the lungful.

High temperatures and humidity accelerate these chemical reactions so the car smells even newer after baking in the hot sun. Don't jump right in and take a big drag, though. Air it out thoroughly and maximize the dilution of off-gassing. If you can, leave your windows open in the garage and crack them a bit when out in the sun so that these dangerous VOCs continue to air out. Roll down your windows while you're driving as well. You'll get some fresh air *and* be able to hear the neighbors *ooh* and *ah* as you roll by in your new car.

vents at the floor level and ceiling level, both of which exhaust to the outside. I put exhaust fans on both vents with a timer set to run automatically at appropriate times during the day. And I turn them on manually when I drive in my car.

It is important that the exhaust fans be on the downwind side of the garage.

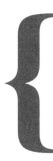

The scent of a new car is the off-gassing of fresh plastics, vinyls, leathers, paints, and synthetic carpets. And new car owners are sucking it down by the lungful.

If you do leave the car windows open in the garage, those new car gasses will be added to the other fumes you want to keep away from your living areas. This is another argument in favor of effectively venting your garage.

You know that film that sometimes builds up on the inside of the windshield? It's from the pollutants your car's air conditioner is pumping in. To get some fresh air, roll down a window or two whenever you can. It's the same rule you apply to your home air quality: The cleaner air is on the outside. Let it in.

A car eventually does decrease its off-gassing. And although our egos may miss that new car smell, our cells will be much happier. And don't fall for the swinging Christmas tree "air freshener" you hang on the rearview mirror

Simple Solution:

Don't set your car's air conditioner or heater to recirculated air. Selecting the outside air option on your dashboard will reduce the number of pollutants you're circulating inside the car.

just inches away from your face. When these fresheners were first marketed, the ads claimed that they "pulled out auto fumes." The original labels also warned consumers to avoid touching the products with your fingers or allow it to touch a painted or plastic surface.

The labeling has been changed, but I'd be surprised if the actual product has. Do you *really* want to breathe something that can damage paint?

What's in a Baby Seat?

I'd known for a while about the dangers of the new car smell, but I learned a few new things after we had Andrew. We innocently purchased what we hoped was the safest car seat and later learned that there's more to safety than protecting against a crash.

Baby car seats also can contain hazardous materials such as antimony, bromine, chlorine, and lead. This is especially troubling because most babies—like Andrew—spend more than just drive-time in that seat. They're lugged around in the carrier at restaurants, stores, and friends' houses, and they're often even left to sleep there.

For more information on healthy car seats for infants, go to www.myhealthyhome.com/carseat.

Fortunately, there are groups that have done testing to help you pick out a less toxic car seat and make certain your child isn't sucking up fumes as he or she dozes.

Do It Yourself—*Safely*

My knowledge about car maintenance goes about as far as jumping a dead battery. But many people like to take care of their cars at home—changing oil, flushing fluids . . . and whatever else it is they do. Yet what mental image comes to mind when you think of an at-home mechanic?

Parts lying around, the smell of oil and gas, a guy in coveralls with his hands covered in grease.

Wait a minute.

We learned in section 3 that we have to be careful about what products we put on our skin. So what about that statement I made earlier, "If you won't drink it, don't put it on your skin"? If you wouldn't consider sipping the oil or grease you use in your car, why would you allow it to sit on your skin, where it can be absorbed into your bloodstream?

Wear gloves when you're working in your garage. Then wash as soon as you're finished, and refrain from using paint thinner, acetone, or other hazardous cleaners to cleanse your hands. These products are likely more toxic than the grease.

Remember, soap and water are your friendliest cleaning agents. Give the extra care and attention to your body that you would to your car.

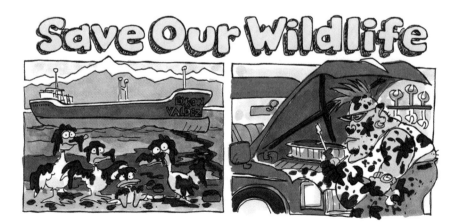

Chapter 13
Going Green
in Your Yard

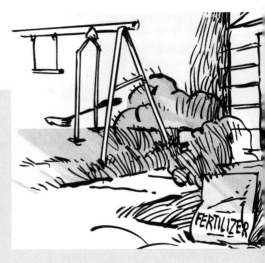

What is it about an unspoiled landscape or any natural setting that's so healing to the human soul? It's not just the great outdoors in a national park that gives us a new lease on life. Even our yards and gardens, regardless of size, offer us the very environment in which we can regroup and find health.

The theologian John Calvin wrote in his book *Institutes* that the earth in all her beauty is similar to a spacious and splendid house, filled with exquisite and abundant furnishings. Like Calvin, we must view our outdoor spaces like we do our homes—as something valuable to protect and pass down to future generations.

And this means not poisoning them.

QUIZ

How Toxic Is Your Home?   Scores

1. How many synthetic pesticides/herbicides do you use around your home and yard?

Anything growing is sprayed	Several	It's pesticide-free
14 pts	7 pts	0 pts

2. How often do you get at least ten minutes outside each day without sunscreen? (Select one)

☐ Daily (0 pts)   ☐ Rarely (5 pts)
☐ A few times a week (1 pt)   ☐ Never (8 pts)

3. Do you pay someone to do your yard work? Yes_____ (5 pts)

4. Do you run in marathons or participate in other types of very strenuous, endurance exercise? Yes_____ (4 pts)

Your "Yard" danger score

1–8	9–16	17–24	25+
Green thumb	Environmentally challenged	Wilting	Agricultural wasteland

Get Out!

Whether we are drawn to mountains, the desert, or the beach, we appreciate the fact that the calm and sense of awe we experience in nature can't be found in our usual surroundings of home and work. When we feel life spiraling out of control or moving too fast, most of us instinctively go find a quiet spot in unspoiled nature. We know that when we get there, we'll be in a place of reprieve and rejuvenation.

In light of the "Living Clean" chapter, we can approach nature with a whole new level of respect. Life is *cleaner* outside. No matter how small the space we employ—even a tiny balcony—escaping from a man-made, four-walled box can do your mind and body good. At the *very* least, open the blinds, throw open a window, and let in some fresh air and sunshine.

Outdoors you will find sunlight, water, air, and soil. Along with food, clothing, and housing, these elements of life are essential to our well-being.

Sunlight

Plants need sunshine to grow, and so do people, both physically and psychologically. In recent years the media has given sunshine a bad rap, warning us to avoid the sun if we want to prevent skin cancer. The truth is that the health benefits of *moderate* exposure to the sun outweighs the risks.

Exposure to the sun causes us to produce vitamin D, and vitamin D is probably the closest thing we have to a miracle vitamin. It's necessary for us to have strong bones and teeth, it regulates the immune system to ward off infections, it helps to prevent certain cancers, and it may even slow the aging process. Working in conjunction with proper nutrition and adequate amounts of sleep, sunlight also triggers the release of serotonin, the neurotransmitter called "the happiness compound" because it promotes a positive mental outlook.

> **Simple Solution:**
> Take a daily vitamin D supplement with at least 2,000 IUs (International Units) during the winter or year-round if you can't get out into the sun each day.

Water

We are watery creatures. Our cells and bodies are 70 percent water. The thousands of chemical reactions in our bodies would not be possible without water. But water sustains us in more ways than through our physiology.

Water appeals to all of our senses. We are drawn to its beauty, we love the sight and sound of it, and as kids we couldn't wait to play in it. We sleep better, work better, and feel better after spending time in or around water. For these reasons, my company's headquarters features a huge indoor waterfall in the lobby. It helps cut down on indoor allergens and acts as a natural humidifier. And workers and visitors report that the sight and sound of it are just plain relaxing.

Air

Okay, so we all know that air is pretty vital to that whole "staying alive" thing. In addition to the simple need to breathe, air provides us with a warning system by carrying the distinctive odors of toxic substances and the sounds of potential danger. It cleans for us, diluting pollutants and moving them from our homes and cities. It also calms us—taking a deep

Ask the Scientist

"Dr. Wentz, can the natural world genuinely help the body heal?"

When I created Sanoviv Medical Institute in Mexico, I deliberately chose a site on a cliff overlooking the Pacific Ocean, away from city pollution and at sea level for maximum oxygen availability.

People have told me that as soon as they enter the gates of Sanoviv they feel the sense of healing begin. Guests experience beautiful sunsets, simple beauty, and serenity all around. They are encouraged to be outside to enjoy the grounds around the medical towers, with the healing salt-water pools, herb gardens, and walkways overlooking the ocean. They can relax surrounded by cooling palm trees and enchanting tropical flowers.

The health benefits of nature are so compelling that many hospitals are restructuring their landscapes to incorporate "healing gardens" and even offer horticultural therapy for patients recovering from stroke or trauma.

One of the reasons nature may be so effective in reducing stress is that it puts the mind in a state similar to meditation. A Japanese study found that people living around trees— even when living in a city—had longer life spans than those living in treeless areas.[2]

breath of fresh air is often the best cure for stress or fear. And as a skydiver and pilot, I can tell you firsthand that air has the power to lift us up, both physically and emotionally.

Soil

Urging his fellow citizens to preserve their farms in the midst of the Great Depression, U.S. President Franklin Delano Roosevelt said, "A nation that destroys its soils destroys itself."[1]

It's true that the six-inch layer of dirt under our feet, warmed by the sun and watered by the rain, is the source of virtually all the energy on the earth. Fertile soil is, of course, much more than just dirt. A square foot of it contains millions of bacteria and thousands of worms and other invertebrates that enrich the soil and make it literally alive. If you have access to even a little plot of soil—whether it's on a window ledge or in a two-acre yard—the best thing you can do is plant something!

Nothing tastes better than vegetables you've grown yourself. Nothing looks brighter than flowers you've planted. And nothing feels more relaxing than sitting under the shade of your own little oxygen-producing tree on a hot summer day.

Don't Be a Pest

Having the benefits of the natural world close by—close enough for us to simply open a door and step out into it—comes at a cost. That's because there are many other organisms—flora and fauna—that are interested in sharing our space, even though we haven't invited them. Often they are also interested in making a meal of the plants that we chose to enhance our homes. And we've got a special name for the unwanted plants and animals that seek to invade a place we've already staked out. We call them pests.

Mankind has been conducting a war against plant and animal pests since we shifted from hunting and gathering to cultivating crops. In the twentieth century the development of synthetic chemicals designed to kill pests—pesticides—became an industry worth billions of dollars every year. After all this time and effort, it's difficult to claim that we're winning, despite our supposed superiority. In fact, at times it appears as if the strategies we most often employ do more harm than good.

First of all, most of our weapons aren't very precise. We use sprays, powders, aerosols, and granules that miss the target more often than not. Over 98 percent of sprayed insecticides and 95 percent of herbicides used today end up somewhere other than the place they were meant to go.[3]

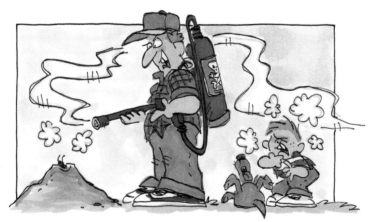

"I'm going to have the healthiest yard in the neighborhood."

Second, we want our poisons to last long enough to do the job, but as a result they remain hazards to our health long after their original purpose has ended. Decades after DDT was banned in the United States and most of the world, it's still being detected in penguins in Antarctica, thousands of miles from where it was used.[4] Persistent organic pollutants such as chlordane—last used twenty years or more ago against termite infestations—can still have carcinogenic effects if the soil where they were deposited is disturbed today.[5]

> Decades after DDT was banned in the United States and most of the world, it's still being detected in penguins in Antarctica, thousands of miles from where it was used.

Third—and far too often—the arsenal we use against pests can only be described as overkill, and too often innocent bystanders pay the price. My brother-in-law learned this valuable lesson a few years ago when he accidentally poisoned his dog while trying to kill slugs and snails in his yard. Fortunately, after intense vomiting and a trip to the veterinary hospital, the dog survived.

Each year, homeowners apply at least ninety million pounds of pesticides to their lawns and gardens. Home use of pesticides rose 42 percent between 1998 and 2001 and now represents the only growth sector of the U.S. pesticide market. And much of this chemical poison doesn't stay outside where we put it. Pesticides applied on residential lawns migrate indoors. Concentrations are often *higher* in house dust than in the soil that surrounds the house, even on farms.[6]

A study by the U.S. Environmental Protection Agency (EPA) found that residues from outdoor pesticides tracked in by pets and on people's shoes can increase the pesticide loads in carpet dust by as much as 400 times.[7]

Pesticides can also persist for years inside homes, where they're not subject to the normal degradation caused by sunlight and rain.

Despite the billions of dollars the agricultural industry spends every year on herbicides, insecticides, rodenticides, and so on, we're still falling behind in this arms race. There are simply too many pests and they are too adaptable to the tools we use against them. Plus, regardless of whatever success we might have in wiping them out in our own yard or garden, reinforcements from elsewhere will quickly replace them.

If we persist in our personal campaign of chemical warfare, we almost surely increase the risk of poisoning ourselves and our families. Pesticides can cause a wide range of health problems, including birth defects, nerve damage, and cancer.[8] Children are especially vulnerable to synthetic pesticides. Their internal organs are still developing, they consume more food and drink per pound of body weight, and they spend much more time playing on floors or lawns, right where the chemicals settle and accumulate.

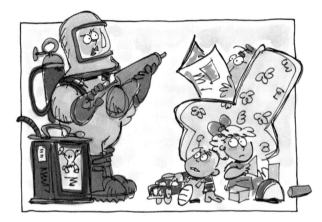

"I think I saw a fly."

All of this because we don't want to share our plants with a bug or we want our lawn to look greener than the neighbor's.

Even a cursory listing of all the toxic substances found in pesticides and their effects on the health of children and other living things would take many pages. On the Internet alone there are more technical resources on the specific hazards that individual pesticides pose than you can possibly use. So here we will focus on some of the things you can do to keep pests under control while avoiding—as much as possible—the use of poisons.

To start, it helps to swallow a small dose of humility and admit that over the past century the use of brute force—nuking the pests with powerful poisons—hasn't worked. With very few exceptions, the goal of eliminating pests has been met with failure. The war never stops escalating, and nature has proven to be every bit as innovative as the scientists in the pesticide industry.

But you *can* get pests under control without endangering the health of your family. The best approach I've seen employs a variety of strategies at the same time so that they achieve a type of synergy that will give you an advantage in overcoming the pests, both plant and animal.

This multipronged plan of attack even has a name—Integrated Pest Management, or IPM.

Integrated Pest Management

Practicing IPM means taking a comprehensive, environmental stance toward the problem of insects, invasive plants, and plant diseases by using a combination of common sense, nontoxic, biological practices. There are several different versions of IPM, most of them focused on industrial-level agriculture, but the principles can be scaled down to be just as effective for personal properties. The principles of IPM, as set by the EPA, include:

Deciding what pest levels are acceptable to you

The emphasis isn't on wiping out every plant and insect you consider a troublemaker but instead keeping them under control. It's impractical as well as impossible to eliminate every pest—you might as well put in AstroTurf and plastic plants and be done with it.

Preventing pests by working with Mother Nature

You begin by taking a comprehensive survey of your property, learning to identify all the plants and animal life that are there, and assessing their health. Then familiarize yourself with the climate and geography of your area. What zone are you in? What are the prevailing temperatures, humidity, and other climatic and geographic conditions?

Ensuring that all the plants you want to keep are healthy

These plants will be your partners in keeping plant pests at bay and resisting animal pests. It helps a lot if your plants suit the growing conditions of your area or—even better—are native to the prevailing conditions.

Obviously, a plant native to Southern California won't do well in a mountain valley in northern Utah. There are people who try to grow tomatoes in their home gardens in Park City, Utah—where the altitude is nearly 7,000 feet, or 2,100 meters—and the venture comes to grief almost every year when the first cold snap comes before the tomatoes are showing more than a tinge of red.

Local garden supply stores will likely have a better supply of plants that naturally call your area home and more information on how to grow them.

Bringing your outdoor areas in line with the local ecosystem can yield major benefits beyond pest control. As part of a major expansion of my company's headquarters in Salt Lake City, we decided to dig up a large expanse of lawn surrounding the building and replace it with xeriscaping, which uses drought-resistant plants. This was an effort to conserve resources, especially water. Due to this change we're saving approximately 750,000 gallons of water every year and making equally dramatic cuts in the use of fertilizer and pesticides. Not only is this good for us, but it's also good for the entire region, which gets less than sixteen inches of precipitation per year.

Identifying and monitoring pests

Once you know what you have on your land, you can make intelligent decisions about what you want to get rid of. Knowledge is power, but you'll want to be careful. There are insects and plants that are good for your lawn and garden, and they can look very similar to the bad guys.

Taking control steps

This is where you part ways with the conventional approaches to pest control. The idea is to form partnerships with certain species of plants and animal life to manage the unwanted weeds, bugs, and diseases. This is also where things get more complicated. But the work is more than worth the long-term results. Among the tactics available are:

Cultivating pest-repelling plants

Rather than poison your garden, lawn, or orchard with pesticides, why not try a simpler, healthier solution? Plant lemon basil with your tomato plants, for example, and you get a combined benefit of better tasting tomatoes while keeping whiteflies away. A peppermint plant will keep ants and mice away.

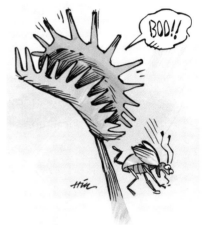

Other insect-repelling plants are rosemary and catnip for mosquito control. The oil from catnip has been found to be many times more effective than DEET. Rosemary, a very popular garden herb, also has an oil that repels mosquitoes. Although rosemary isn't very hardy in cold climates, you can grow it in a pot and take it inside for the winter.

Marigolds have a particular odor that many insects find objectionable. They are good plants for repelling mosquitoes as well as aphids and other insects that can attack vegetable crops. One downside in considering marigolds is that their "fragrance" often isn't pleasing to humans, either.

Calling in the bug patrol

There are good bugs and bad bugs. The bad bugs eat everything you are trying to grow in your yard and garden, and the good bugs eat the bad bugs. Actually, many of the insects you can enlist don't do the search and destroy work themselves. They devote their lives to enjoying the nectar and pollen from your flowers and creating babies. It's the larvae of these offspring that do the actual hunting and eating of the harmful bugs. Insects that can help with specific problems include:

- Ladybugs (Ladybird beetles) are effective against aphids, scale insects, mealybugs, and mites.
- Green lacewings **larvae** (aphid lions) combat infestations of spider mites, thrips, leafhoppers, whiteflies. and caterpillar eggs.

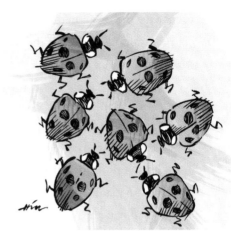

- Praying mantis are as ferocious as they look if you are a pest insect within striking distance. The nymphs begin preying on insects as small as mosquitoes as soon as they hatch in the spring.
- Syrphid flies eat aphids and serve as valuable pollinators.

Go to www.myhealthyhome.com/bugs to learn more about all the good bugs you may want to welcome into your yard.

You can invite friendly insects to your garden by growing plants and flowers that provide food and shelter for them. When you purchase good bugs at a nursery or garden center, make sure that you have an adequate amount of plants that provide their food supply. Some of the plants you'll want as food sources are caraway, coriander clover, dill, alyssum, nasturtiums, and fennel.

Bringing in the birds

Most pests in our yard or garden have native predators we can turn into our allies. With their high metabolism and energy needs, insect-eating birds are champions at consuming insect pests. Swallows, wrens, and warblers live primarily on insects, larvae, and insect eggs, but nearly all of the birds that visit your yard or garden—even hummingbirds—help to keep insect pests under control. And if you want to make your yard friendly to insectivorous birds or beneficial insects, the first step is a no-brainer: Don't use synthetic chemical pesticides.

Maintaining and adding to diversity

When we build new homes, we may start with a piece of semiwild, undeveloped land that has something like two hundred different species of plants, along with all the associated insects, worms, and other invertebrates

> { If you want to make your yard friendly to insectivorous birds or beneficial insects, the first step is a no-brainer: Don't use synthetic chemical pesticides. }

that have inhabited the area since time immemorial. Often we replace all this diversity with one species of grass, a few shrubs, and flowers—probably none of them native. As a result, we are disappointed when the place looks bleak and uninviting, and we have to spend massive time, effort, and money trying to force our garden to grow.

Simple Solution:

Plant a large, diverse range of plants in your yard—native species are best. The more the merrier, and healthier.

Seeking out alternatives to synthetic poisons

There are many little tricks you can use to control pests, and they don't involve hazardous chemicals. For example, if you're trying to get tough, deeply rooted weeds out from cracks in the driveway, sidewalk, or patio, pour some boiling water from a

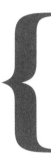

Go to www.myhealthyhome.com/ipm for more nontoxic gardening tips and resources.

kettle and watch them wilt and die like the Wicked Witch of the West in *The Wizard of Oz*.

The Pesticide Action Network offers a wealth of information on alternatives to synthetic pesticides, and the U.S. Environmental Protection Agency provides many resources to help with IPM—and don't forget the experts at your local gardening center.

Using biological pesticides

An important component of IPM is the use of biological pesticides, or biopesticides. This is one area of IPM in which you will almost certainly need some expert guidance. Biopesticides are products derived from natural sources including bacteria, fungi, and viruses. The use of such traditional remedies as garlic, mint, and baking soda could be considered early biopesticides as well.

My sister recently introduced me to NoLo bait, which is made from flaky wheat bran. The spores affect only grasshoppers and closely related insects, so she can be the one who gets to eat her healthy veggies, instead of the grasshoppers.

> Visit www.myhealthyhome.com/biopesticides for additional information.

Integrated Pest Management is a reaction to the mindset that became prevalent with the development of modern synthetic pesticides in the mid-1940s. We thought we had developed "silver bullets" that would solve all our agricultural problems. We know better now.

Perhaps the most significant aspect of IPM is the potential for reducing health hazards for you and your family. In fact, many practitioners of IPM consider reducing the use of pesticides as the most important goal of this approach, ahead even of effective pest control itself.

IPM has many similarities to Dr. Wentz's approach to nutrition—his insistence that supplements contain all the necessary ingredients in the right amount and correct balance. If we can achieve that right mix of natural elements—water, air, fertilizers, pollinators, and so on—in our yards and gardens, we'll have nature working *for* us instead of against us.

Get Physical!

Being outdoors—watching sunsets or stars and taking in lovely landscapes—is one of the best health tonics I know.

However, even better than observing the outdoors is working in it. Working in your pesticide-free yard is a good start. And one simple way of improving your outlook, instilling a good dose of both wonder and humility, is planting seeds in the ground and seeing them turn into living, growing organisms. Your body, mind, and spirit will reap the benefits. This is also a great opportunity for family time as you do chores in the yard or tend a garden together.

Watching the seeds sprout is just the beginning. In just a couple of months they become—through what seems like nothing short of a miracle— food that will nourish your cells and taste so much better than anything you could buy at the grocery store.

Outdoor exercise is also much better than mindlessly wishing that the minutes would go by faster while sweating on the treadmill. Studies have shown that physical exertion involved in digging, tilling, planting, weeding, fertilizing, and harvesting is positively linked to bone mineral density, sleep quality, hand strength, muscle tone, and psychological well-being.

A daily routine of working in a garden will keep at bay heart disease, obesity, high blood pressure, adult-onset diabetes, osteoporosis, and stroke. A critical component for maintaining physical fitness is weight-bearing exercise, and for that you can't beat carrying watering cans, pushing a wheelbarrow, or turning a compost pile. And focusing on the health of other living things can be a sort of meditation, both pleasurable and mind sharpening. It's another reason to swap your elliptical for a set of garden tools.

Work Works Wonders

Say *that* three times fast . . .

Physical work has become inconvenient in our hip, technology-driven lifestyles, so we now need to look for daily opportunities to move our bodies. Yet there are a lot of simple ways to get a workout without seriously disrupting our daily routines:

- Parking at the back of the lot
- Taking the stairs rather than the elevator
- Handling our own luggage

Taken together, these basic exercises will yield life-altering cumulative benefits.

Fifty years ago, humans burned about seven hundred more calories every day than we do now.[9] We've minimized our calorie output by engineering the basic manual activities—from rolling down car windows to mowing the grass—out of our lives. The machines are now doing our work for us, but we can begin burning those calories again by taking advantage of the

{ Fifty years ago, humans burned about seven hundred more calories every day than we do now...machines are now doing our work for us. }

spare five or ten minutes we all have a few times every day. Studies show that three ten-minute walks burn calories and enhance health nearly as effectively as a single thirty-minute stroll.[10]

Play = Long Life

What's pointless and easily replaced?

Play.

Or that's what we've come to believe. Yet research is proving that happy, entertaining relationships literally change the biochemistry of our brains for the better, whereas loneliness raises our risk of high blood pressure, depression, and an early death.

A little fun at the end of the day has great benefits for kids, too. Researchers from the University of Bristol measured the activity of 5,500 twelve-year-olds and found that just fifteen minutes a day spent doing moderate physical activity—like playing tag in the backyard—will reduce the likelihood of being obese by up to 50 percent.[11]

So have some fun! Build a fort or have a pillow fight with your kids. Everyone will reap the benefits.

Going for Gold

For those of you who take physical activity to the extreme, running marathons, biking for miles and miles, or pumping serious weights in the gym, it's best to remember that strenuous exercise puts a lot of wear and tear on your cells. During high-impact workouts, your body is producing and expending energy—and creating free radicals through oxidation.

Your body generally has no problem handling the daily grind. But when you're pushing your body to the limit, you'll need some extra antioxidant protection. This is especially true if your body is compromised by an illness or if you are under a lot of psychological stress.

And marathon runners already know about the toll it can take on the knees. If you participate in sports in which your joints sustain frequent significant impacts, be sure to take a supplement such as glucosamine to give your body what it needs to continually replace and strengthen that important cushion of cartilage in your joints. Professional athletes know that it's the knees that go first, so do what you can to keep them functional.

My sister, Julie, lives in a small town in southern Utah where an ordinance requires that residents control their outdoor lights—by shielding them, pointing them directly toward a building or ground, or shutting them off altogether—so residents can enjoy the full splendor of the night sky.

So many of us now live in towns and cities filled with light pollution from street lights, twenty-four-hour convenience stores, and never-ending traffic. We forget just how awe inspiring it is to look up and *really* see the moon and stars.

Although I'm not fortunate enough to live in an area that mandates "dark hours," I've found that there are many ways to reconnect with the natural world. Reneé and I have surrounded our home with plants and trees, inside and out. And we take full advantage of the natural places close to our home. For me, there is nothing more rejuvenating than skiing or biking through the trees in the Wasatch Mountains of Utah.

It's on those great sunshine-drenched white powder snow days that I'm reminded of the Greek myth of the giant Antaeus. According to the legend, he would challenge all passersby to wrestling matches. He was unbelievably strong as long as he remained in contact with his Mother Earth.

The Greek hero Hercules encountered Antaeus, who challenged him to wrestle. Despite his strength and skill, Hercules could not defeat the giant— every time he threw Antaeus to the ground the giant sprang up, stronger than before. Then the goddess Athena whispered Antaeus's secret in Hercules's ear, and Hercules grabbed Antaeus in a bear hug and held him off the ground. Antaeus's strength steadily ebbed away, and Hercules crushed him in his arms.

Whenever I've spent too many days in a row in my office or on airplanes, I know that, like Antaeus, I need to reconnect with the earth to be at my best. But part of accepting this valuable connection is the responsibility to do what I can to keep the earth clean. That's why protecting the planet through recycling, conservation, and reducing pollutants is so important.

And our homes are the perfect place to start.

What Simple Solutions will you add to your Garage and Yard?

Scores

1. I will: (Select all that apply)

   ☐ Finish and seal any drywall, ductwork, electric wiring, and seams in the garage walls and ceiling (8 pts)

   ☐ Install a fan in the garage to remove polluted air (10 pts)

   ☐ Properly dispose of any of the dangerous chemical products like pesticides, paints, and motor fluids that may be currently stored in the garage (5 pts for half; 10 pts for all)

   ☐ Seal any remaining paint cans by placing plastic wrap under the lid and turning it upside down (2 pts)

   ☐ Move any small gas-powered devices out of the garage and into a separate shed or storage area (4 pts)

   ☐ Park the car outside the garage or leave the garage door open whenever possible (4 pts)

2. I will: (Select all that apply)

   ☐ Always wear gloves when working on the car (5 pts)

   ☐ Wash hands with soap and water, not paint thinner, when finished working in the garage (3 pts)

3. I will: (Select all that apply)

   ☐ Get at least a few minutes of daily sunshine without sunscreen (8 pts)

   ☐ Take a vitamin D supplement in the winter or when I can't get outside (8 pts)

   ☐ Add plants indoors as natural air fresheners (4 pts)

   ☐ Add a water feature, such as a miniature waterfall or fountain, to my living area (4 pts)

4. I will: (Select all that apply)

   ☐ Trade in use of pesticides and herbicides for a more integrated approach to controlling pests (15 pts)

   ☐ If continuing use of pesticides or herbicides, commit to read the labels carefully and take precautions to protect family and pets (4 pts)

   ☐ Learn what native plants in my area are good for pest control (5 pts)

   ☐ Ask my yard-care company and/or neighbors about what pest control treatments they use (3 pts)

   ☐ Replace non-native plants in the yard with hardier, native species (2 pts for each new species)

   ☐ Plant natural pest-repelling plants like lemon basil, rosemary, catnip, and marigolds (1 pt for each)

   ☐ Add a bird feeder or other bird-friendly feature to my yard to naturally reduce bugs (4 pts)

   ☐ Add more types of plant life to the yard (1 pt for each)

Your Simple Solutions positive score:	
Your "Garage" danger score:	-
Your "Yard" danger score:	-
Your Garage and Yard Health total:	

Are you making a positive difference?

Epilogue One

Over the past few decades, I've worked closely alongside my father on many projects that were huge in scope. Together we've formulated new products, taken our company global, and helped change many lives along the way. But somehow this relatively finite project—this book—has had great personal significance.

Working on something this creative and personal has illuminated our similarities and differences. Like most fathers and sons, we share certain physical features and have common interests, but there are many ways in which we live in two distinct worlds. I worked on my portion of the book on my laptop or iPhone, usually in an airport or hotel room. My father wrote most of his contributions by hand, using a good, old-fashioned no. 2 pencil. I drew from my very recent experience of "cleaning house" for the birth of my first child. Meanwhile, my father looked back on a lifetime of professional and personal discoveries that he had long since put into practice in his own life.

You might say that one of us represents the past and the other the present. But this book came about because both of us are determined to have an impact on the future. Where else could we focus our efforts? Those most vulnerable to serious and lasting damage from a toxic environment are also the world's most precious resource—our children. Like my dad did for me, I will strive to ensure a healthy and happy life for Andrew—and the daughter Reneé and I just welcomed into the world.

Sure, I could feel defeated by the constant bombardment of new technologies, new drugs, and new products that threaten to make our lives shorter. But I feel incredible hope in the increasing awareness among people everywhere of the true cost of convenience and the growing tide of individuals and families who are ready to take action to defend their long-term wellness. The many conversations I had while writing the book opened my eyes to just how many parents and grandparents out there share my concerns. The idea of a community standing together to create change on a larger scale strengthened my hope for the future.

History has taught us that concerned citizens can be a powerful force for meaningful change. But as I learned with the birth of my first child, the actions that can have the most impact are often simple ones—changes we can make as individuals in our own homes. There's no need to wait for a lumbering government or timid corporate sector to come around. You have the power today to make a long-term impact on the health of your loved ones.

Feeling overwhelmed?

I was, too, until I realized that, although I couldn't change the world in just a few years for my family, I could change the most important place in their world—our home. We have a choice to make when we become aware of dangers: Be frightened or take action. I hope you'll choose the latter by concentrating on the solutions from this book that are within your reach. Don't get hung up on huge projects that you can't afford or areas that intimidate you.

It's okay to start small.

In fact, simple is usually best. That's why I love the short but profound "to do" list written by newspaper columnist Mary Schmich in 1997 for college graduates. It started with the simple phrase, "Wear sunscreen."

I've written my own version below, which I hope will be fun and useful for those of you who are starting out on a quest to achieve a less toxic life.

Ladies and Gentlemen of the Twenty-First Century

Wear gloves.

If I could give you just one bit of advice it would be to wear gloves. Whether you're scrubbing the floors, poisoning your yard, or changing the oil in your car, just remember, if you wouldn't drink it, don't touch it.

Enjoy the taste of color. Never mind that color doesn't taste. Enjoy the beauty of colorful foods that nourish your cells.

Drink bottled water when you travel, but protect your plastic container.

Drink purified water when you're home, but change your filters often. Drink lots of water. Travel.

Don't mess too much with your skin, or by the time you're forty, it will look eighty.

Enjoy the power and beauty of your skin cells. Ignore the tantalizing marketing of cosmetic companies trying to cover, color, and contaminate your natural appearance. You probably won't understand the power and beauty of your skin until it's wrinkled and faded. You are beautiful just the way you are.

But lose the weight. Trust me, in twenty years you'll look back at photos and recall how much more life you had when there was much less of you.

Open a window.

Breathe.

Don't worry about your family's health. Or worry, but know that it's your choices that most often decide the outcome. Worrying only adds stress, which reduces your odds if you're rolling the dice and living by chance. Don't gamble.

The Gauss meter reveals, the mold dog barks, and your nose knows.

Share your world. Bugs may be pests, but they don't pester like your spouse and your kids, and you keep them around.

Don't be reckless with pesticides. Don't live near people who are reckless with theirs.

Fluoride kills. Floss instead.

Lose the silver fillings. Keep your beautiful memories.

Don't feel guilty for damage already done. Do one extra thing every day that brings health to your home and family.

Open another window.

Breathe.

Don't waste your money on dryer sheets. Sometimes your socks will stick to your pajamas. It's okay.

Your nose knows. Smell nothing and smell it often.

Log off.

Get plenty of rest. These days it's the only time you're not too busy to dream.

Maybe you have children, maybe you don't. Take off your shoes anyway.

You never know who will use the ten-second rule to eat something that fell on the floor.

Trust your instincts. Don't forget that other "sense" that is incredibly powerful—common sense.

Open all the windows.

Breathe.

Don't worry about the future. Change it. Today, I offer you solutions. Some proven, some theory, but all with good intentions. If I miss the mark on some and they are not life saving, trust that they will not harm you.

Build your immune system, not Big Pharma's pockets. Only one has your best interests at heart.

Simplify.

Don't poison your house to kill a fly. Bug strips will show you who's not paying rent.

Get to know the way of life your parents had when they were kids. Your parents' past holds the key to your children's healthy future.

Research.

Accept certain inalienable but simple truths: Your home and car are polluted. You can change that.

Respect warning labels. Better yet, don't use products that require them.

Are all the windows open?

Breathe.

Science cannot move quickly enough to ensure product safety. Look out for yourself and your family. You are responsible. When you point in blame, three fingers point back at you.

Learn.

Be careful whose advice you buy. Be the type of person who has learned to question. I hope you'll question my suggestions and do some research. Find answers for yourself. When you can't find answers, stop, think, and do what your gut tells you. Do it for our children's future.

But trust me on the gloves.

—Dave Wentz

Epilogue Two

Modern society is in the midst of the greatest scientific experiment in history. We are exposing our young people to a world full of toxins, without any idea of how their health and well-being are affected. Again and again we release newly invented toxins into our air, water, soil, and consumer products. When the experiment goes bad—when we learn that exposure is causing serious harm—we look back and wonder why tests weren't performed to make sure the chemical was safe for humans and other living things.

A new chemical substance is discovered about every nine seconds during the workday. Chemists discovered the eighteen millionth chemical substance known to science on June 15, 1998. Many thousands more have been developed since then. Most of these substances are of little use, but thousands are incorporated into consumer products or industrial processes every year.[1]

The public has no way of knowing whether a large majority of the chemicals in the greatest abundance present hazards to their health—or the health of their children. There is no way to know how serious the health risks could be or even whether those chemicals are under control.[2] We may know other things about them—that they prevent tomatoes from spoiling or that they kill insects, for example—but we don't know what effects they may have on human cells or human bodies. If those effects don't show up for a long time, we may be making the toxins part of our environment for years or decades.

The serious problems come from the fact that everyone is being exposed—there are no controls. Everybody who breathes the air, drinks the water, or eats the food grown in the soil is included in the test group. When we finally become aware of long-term negative effects, millions of people will have been effected.

Although none of us escape the threats our society poses to our health, there are many reasons why we should place special emphasis on the young when discussing environmental health. They range from the purely emotional—why my son and I first considered writing this book—to strictly scientific—our understanding of how much more vulnerable the fetus, infant, and child are compared to the adult human.

The exposures that pose threats to children's health begin even before conception. Any toxic chemicals that may have accumulated in a woman's body may cross the placenta and affect the embryo or fetus during critical periods of development. Most toxic chemicals, such as pesticides, are fat-soluble and can build up in fat tissues in the body. The prospective mother's body mobilizes her nutritional and energy reserves to provide the fetus with the best nutrition possible, but toxic chemicals can go along for the ride, accumulating in the fetus instead.

Even after birth, children's detoxification mechanisms are underdeveloped and unable to fully protect them from chemicals. Children also breathe faster and eat and drink more in proportion to their bodyweight compared to adults. The result is greater exposure to chemicals from the same air, food, and water.

There is absolutely no doubt that toxic elements completely surround us in today's world. We cannot deny that the environmental influences on our health—especially the health of the younger portions of our society—have become not just a major concern but in fact the most important health problem in the world today.

I've shared these concerns many times in conversations with friends, colleagues, and even strangers on airplanes. Often they ask, "If it's really that bad, is there even any hope for us?" I always answer with an emphatic "Yes!" By controlling what you and your family breathe, eat, and drink as well as what you permit to be in your surroundings, you'll be protecting and fostering life itself. By increasing cellular defenses through optimal nutrition, you will be better able to fight the toxins you cannot avoid. By tending to your closest universe, you will bring change to the world.

I cannot believe that we were put here to succumb to something as mindless as the fact that humans are turning the world into a toxic cradle. We may not be able to bar all the dangers that threaten to invade, but we can protect this universe within. By starting from the inside out, we change the bigger picture. Caring for yourself and those you love will protect not only your family but also the future of the planet.

One of the questions I've often asked myself—and regularly posed to my children—is this: Are you living by choice or by chance? Are you passively hoping your health, happiness, or life itself will turn out well, or are you actively engaged in achieving the results you desire? Certainly there are circumstances for which we have no control. Yet it's far too easy for us to dismiss nearly every outcome in life as unavoidable.

Of all the wisdom I have gained in my seven decades of life, the most important is the knowledge that health and time are two precious assets that we rarely recognize or appreciate until they have been depleted. As with time, health is the raw material of life. You can use it wisely or waste it or even kill it. To accomplish all that we are capable of, we would need a hundred lifetimes. If we had forever in our mortal lives, we would have no need to adjust our lifestyle habits, set goals, plan effectively, or set priorities. We could squander our time and health and perhaps still manage to realize our dreams, if only by chance.

Yet in reality, we're given only one lifespan on earth to do our earthly best. We must choose.

Choosing optimal health is the dream I have for my children, their children, and yours. May you love life and live it to its fullest in happiness and health.

—Dr. Myron Wentz

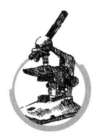

Acknowledgments

To all those named and unnamed who have contributed to the success of this project. We remain profoundly grateful to each of you who have had an impact on our professional and personal journeys.

To our coauthor, Donna Wallace. Thank you for your patience and persistence, especially in chasing us around the world for interviews and interaction.

To everyone at Vanguard Press for giving this project a much larger life. Special thanks to Roger Cooper as well as Georgina Levitt, Amanda Ferber, and Cisca Schreefel for their guidance, enthusiasm, and down-to-earth approach. Stephen Saffel also deserves our gratitude for greatly improving the manuscript with his insightful questions and thorough edits.

To Amy Haran, whose dedication to this project and tireless ability to bring our thoughts to life made this work possible. To Peter Van Duser for his depth of research, inquisitive mind, and attention to scientific documentation.

Kevin Guest, we offer you our greatest appreciation for spearheading our vision and making it a reality. Jeff Yates, we're still amazed at our good fortune of hiring a financial officer who just happened to know the ins and outs of the publishing industry. Your expertise (and good humor) was essential.

Thanks also to Denis Waitley, Tony Jeary, Lyle MacWilliam, Dr. Michael B. White, Dr. Ray Strand, Michael Scott, and the staff at Sanoviv Medical Institute for their valuable feedback and contributions.

To Nathan Parét and John Cordova for delivering a ridiculously time-intensive and creative layout. To Pat Hill and Val Bagley for enlivening the book with their illustrations and cartoons.

To Diane Leroy and Melissa Fields for providing the necessary encouragement (and threats) to keep two constantly distracted authors and their teams on task. To Kim Pratt and Ashley Collins for serving as sounding boards and dedicating their time and talents to marketing and promotions.

And to the many other women—coworkers, customers, friends, and family members—who took the time to read the manuscript and offer their keen insights and challenging questions.

Finally, to Reneé and Prudence, our biggest fans and toughest critics. It's remarkable that you put up with our nonsense during a normal year. That you supported us for months of collaborative writing is a miracle for which we will always be grateful.

We also offer our special thanks to the following people, who provided early support for this book and its message. Your enthusiasm was essential to our success.

Lisa Ng and Ivan Wong
Susanne and John Cunningham
Sophia Marcoux and Jacques Fiset
April and Mike Fano
Collette Larsen and Zachary Ross
Tom and Lorie Mulhern
Bill Ohochinsky and
    Donna Thrasher
Heshie Segal
Deanna and David Waters
Majid and Kahnoush Mokhbery
John and Anne Northrup
Barbara Souther
Pete and Dora Zdanis
Lynn Allen-Johnson
Owen and Marcie Briles
Dan and Rebecca Brink
Simon and Kelly Chan
Dan and Nanc Christy
David and Tricia Delevante
Faye and Raymond Despins
Paul and Ellen Dueck
J'en El and
    Michael Adamson, Ph.D.

Brett and Melanie Ethridge
Dana and Paul Ethridge
Theresa Haney and
    Pepi Diaz-Salazar
Michael and Barbara Hollender
Penny and Phil Kirk
Arnie and Linda Knight
Paul and Leslee Maki
Mike and Miriam Miller
Janet L. Moore
Mario and Elia Ray
Karen and Tim Shumka
Susan Waitley
Rick and Terri Young
Seta Der Artinian and
    Hubert Krause
Line and Luc Dubois
Jean-Pierre Gagné and
    Nicole Boulé
Rita Hui
Michel and Suzanne Lavoie
Isabelle Wilson

Acknowledgments

John and Patty Abraham
Daryl and Robert Allen
Bud and Bunny Barth
Brian, Jaclyn, Dylan, and
    Landri Bohlke
Chris and Helen Bolton-Jamieson
Larry and Nancy Bunn
Gene and Gwen Burnell,
    Todd, Garrett, and Whitney
Michael Callejas
Mable and Vincent Chan
Dean and Sherri Chionis and
    Matt Chionis
Sheila and Garry Dancho
Tony and Tammy Daum
Barbara and Dr. Norman Dawson
Claude and Maryse DuQuette
Robin Ellis
Jim and Dian Fawver
Dustin and Melissa Fields
Barbara Fonger
Leanne Grechulk
Dr. Steve and Andrea Hryszczuk
Daniel and Dr. Paige Hunter
Fiona Jamieson-Folland and
    Chris Folland

Rory Jones
Jordan Kemper
Dr. Deborah Kern
Dean and Evelyn Koontz
Lyne and Germain Lafortune
Elaine Lee
Ri Yue Liu
Carmen Marshall
Dixie Moore
Aaron Dinh and Cathy Ngo
Gene and Sandra Onley
Liza Pascal and Ayan Rivera
Peter and Bibiana Pau
Sven and Patricia Poulsen
Annette and Victor Que
Patti Roney
Justina Rudez
Matt, Shanna, Will and Ava Ryan
Lloyd and Nikki Singer
Dwight and Karen Spaulding
Brian and Amber Thiel
Duke and Sheila Tubtim
Dr. Karen Wolfe
Terry and Terri Wright
Dr. Wen Chi Wu and
    Zang Houng Wu

About the Authors

Dave Wentz

Dave Wentz is chief executive officer of USANA Health Sciences, a state-of-the-art manufacturer of nutritional supplements and health products. He received a bachelor's degree in bioengineering from the University of California, San Diego. Dave lives with his wife, Reneé, and children, Andrew and Sydney, in Salt Lake City, Utah, where he enjoys skydiving, playing volleyball and soccer, mountain biking, and skiing Utah's famous powder.

Myron Wentz, Ph.D.

Dr. Myron Wentz holds a Ph.D. in microbiology with a specialty in immunology from the University of Utah. He founded Gull Laboratories in 1974 and developed the first commercially available diagnostic test for the Epstein-Barr virus. Later he founded USANA Health Sciences and Sanoviv Medical Institute. Dr. Wentz was honored in June 2007 with the Albert Einstein Award for Outstanding Achievement in the Life Sciences. He is the author of *A Mouth Full of Poison* and *Invisible Miracles*. He travels the world with his lovely partner, Prudence.

Donna K. Wallace

Donna K. Wallace has penned fifteen books with accomplished speakers, physicians, therapists, and celebrities. Her recent projects include *The Creation Health Breakthrough* (Hachette, 2007) with Dr. Monica Reed as well as the international best-selling book *What Your Doctor Doesn't Know About Nutritional Medicine May Be Killing You* (Thomas Nelson, 2000) with Dr. Ray Strand. Donna and her family live in Bozeman, Montana.

Notes

THE BEDROOM: CHAPTER 1

1. U.S. Centers for Disease Control, Agency for Toxic Substances and Disease Registry, "Public Health Statement for Antimony," CAS# 7440–36–0, December 1992, http://www.atsdr.cdc.gov/phs/phs.asp?id=330&tid=58 (accessed June 10, 2010).

2. L. Birnbaum and D. Staskal, "Brominated Flame Retardants: Cause for Concern?" *Environmental Health Perspectives*, 112 (2004) 9-17.

3. SixWise.com, "The 6+ Synthetic Fabrics You Most Want to Avoid and Why," http://www.sixwise.com/newsletters/05/12/21/the-6-synthetic-fabrics-you-most-want-to-avoid-and-why.htm (accessed January 2, 2009).

4. Croplife Foundation, "Pesticide Use in U.S. Crop Production: 2002," http://www.croplifefoundation.org/Documents/PUD/NPUD%202002/Fung%20&%20Herb%202002%20Data%20Report.pdf (accessed June 29, 2010).

5. Fragranced Products Information Network, "Background," http://www.fpinva.org/text/1a5d908–117.html (accessed January 19, 2010); June Russell's Health Facts, "Chemical Sensitivities and Perfumes," http://www.jrussellshealth.org/chemsensperf.html (accessed January 8, 2010).

6. K. Leong, "Is Perfume Toxic to Your Health?" *Associated Content: Health and Wellness*, August 14, 2008, http://www.associatedcontent.com/article/929891/is_perfume_toxic_to_your_health.html?cat=5 (accessed January 7, 2010).

7. Institute of Medicine, "Clearing the Air: Asthma and Indoor Air Exposures," *Indoor Chemical Exposures*, ch. 6, 247–50 (Washington, D.C.: National Academy Press, 2000).

8. H. Scott et al., "Steroidgenesis in the Fetal Testis and Its Susceptibility to Disruption by Exogenous Compounds," *Endocrine Reviews* 30, (2009): 883–925.

9. Canadian Centre for Occupational Health and Safety "Health Effects of Acetone," December 1997, http://www.ccohs.ca/oshanswers/chemicals/chem_profiles/acetone/health_ace.html#_1_9 (accessed January 8, 2010).

10. N. Soukaseum, "Determining the Toxicity Level of Perfumes and Colognes," Project No. J1431, California State Fair, 2006, Project Abstract, http://www.usc.edu/CSSF/History/2006/Panels/J14.html#J1431 (accessed July 1, 2010).

11. California Environmental Protection Agency Air Resources Board, "California Dry Cleaning Industry Technical Assessment Report," August 2005, http://www.arb.ca.gov/toxics/dryclean/draftdrycleantechreport.pdf (accessed December 21, 2009).

12. K. W. Thomas et al., "Effect of Dry-cleaned Clothes on Tetrachloroethylene Levels in Indoor Air, Personal Air, and Breath for Residents of Several New Jersey Homes," *Journal of Exposure Analysis and Environmental Epidemiology* 1, no. 4 (October 1991): 475–90.

13. L. M. Langan and S. M. Watkins, "Pressure of Menswear on the Neck in Relation to Visual Performance," *Human Factors* 29 (1987): 67–71.

14. C. Teng et al., "Effect of a Tight Necktie on Intraocular Pressure," *British Journal of Ophthalmology* 87 (2003): 946–48.

15. E. Brown, "Tight-pants Syndrome: Cause of Abdominal Pressure," The Free Library, http://www.thefreelibrary.com/%22Tight-pants+syndrome.%22+%28cause+of+abdominal+pressure%29-a017104523 (accessed June 29, 2010).

16. N. I. Jowett and C. G. F. Robinson, "The Tight Pants Syndrome—A Sporting Variant," *Postgraduate Medical Journal* 72 (1996): 239–40.

17. S. Lunder and A. Jacob, "Fire Retardants in Toddlers and Their Mothers," Environmental Working Group, http://www.ewg.org/reports/pbdesintoddlers (accessed March 31, 2010); ToxFAQs™ (U.S. Centers for Disease Control, Agency for Toxic Substances & Disease Registry), "ToxFAQs™ for Polybrominated Diphenyl Ethers," September 2004, http://www.atsdr.cdc.gov/tfacts68-pbde.html (accessed March 31, 2010).

THE BEDROOM: CHAPTER 2

1. M. Munowitz, *Knowing: The Nature of Physical Law* (New York: Oxford University Press, 2005).

2. N. Werthheimer and E. Leeper, "Electrical Wiring Configurations and Childhood Cancer," *American Journal of Epidemiology* 109 (1979) 273-84.

3. Scientific Committee on Emerging and Newly Identified Health Risks (SCENIHR), "Health Effects of Exposure to EMF," 2009, Brussels, Belgium.

4. World Health Organization, "What Are Electromagnetic Fields?" http://www.who.int/peh-emf/about/WhatisEMF/en/ (accessed October 1, 2009); Energex, "Effects of EMFs—Do EMFs Cause Adverse Health Effects?" http://www.energex.com.au/network/emf/community_emf_approach.html (accessed October 1, 2009).

5. J. M. Delgado, J. Leal, J. L. Monteagudo, and M. G. Gracia, "Embryological Changes Induced by Weak, Extremely Low Frequency Electromagnetic Fields," *Journal of Anatomy* 134, pt. 3 (May 1982): 533–51; J. D. Harland and R. P. Liburdy, "Environmental Magnetic Fields Inhibit the Antiproliferative Action of Tamoxifen and Melatonin in a Human Breast Cancer Cell Line," *Bioelectromagnetics* 18, no. 8 (1997): 555–62; O. Johansson, "Disturbance of the Immune System by Electromagnetic Fields: A Potentially Underlying Cause for Cellular Damage and Tissue Repair Reduction which Could Lead to Disease and Impairment," *Pathophysiology* 16, nos. 2–3 (2009): 157–77; R. Meinert and J. Michaelis, "Meta-analyses of Studies on the Association between Electromagnetic Fields and Childhood Cancer," *Radiation and Environmental Biophysics* 35, no. 1 (1996): 11–18; M. Otto and K. E. von Muhlendahl, "Electromagnetic Fields (EMF): Do They Play a Role in Children's Environmental Health (CEH)?" *International Journal of Hygiene and Environmental Health* 210, no. 5 (2007): 635–44; D. A. Savitz, "Overview of Epidemiologic Research on Electric and Magnetic Fields and Cancer," *American Industrial Hygiene Association Journal* 54, no. 4 (1993): 197–204.

6. Otto and von Muhlendahl, "Electromagnetic Fields"; N. Wertheimer and E. Leeper, "Electrical Wiring Configurations and Childhood Cancer," *American Journal of Epidemiology* 109, no. 3 (1979): 273–84.

7. Wertheimer and Leeper, "Electrical Wiring Configurations and Childhood Cancer."

8. T. Tynes, L. Klaeboe, and T. Haldorsen, "Residential and Occupational Exposure to 50 Hz Magnetic Fields and Malignant Melanoma: A Population Based Study," *Occupational and Environmental Medicine* 60, no. 5 (2003): 343–47.

9. M. Feychting et al., "Occupational Magnetic Field Exposure and Neurodegenerative Disease," *Epidemiology* 14, no. 4 (2003): 413–19; N. Hakansson et al., "Neurodegenerative Diseases in Welders and Other Workers Exposed to High Levels of Magnetic Fields," *Epidemiology* 14, no. 4 (2003): 420–26.

10. G. M. Lee et al., "A Nested Case-control Study of Residential and Personal Magnetic Field Measures and Miscarriages," *Epidemiology* 13, no.1 (2002): 21–31; D. K. Li and R. R. Neutra, "Magnetic Fields and Miscarriage," *Epidemiology* 13 no. 2, (2002): 237–38; Y. N. Cao, Y. Zhang, and Y. Liu, "Effects of Exposure to Extremely Low Frequency Electromagnetic Fields on Reproduction of Female Mice and Development of Offsprings," *Zhonghua Lao Dong Wei Sheng Zhi Ye Bing Za Zhi* 24 no. 8 (2006): 468–70.

11. A. Goldsworthy, "The Dangers of Electromagnetic Smog," *h.e.s.e Project: Human Ecological Social Economic*, 2007, under "EM Fields" and "Papers," http://www.hese-project.org/hese-uk/en/papers/electrosmog_dangers.pdf (accessed January 26, 2010); A. Goldsworthy, "The Biological Effects of Weak Electromagnetic Fields," *h.e.s.e Project: Human Ecological Social Economic*, 2007, under "EM Fields" and "Papers," http://www.hese-project.org/hese-uk/en/papers/goldsworthy_bio_weak_em_07.pdf (accessed January 26, 2010).

THE BEDROOM: CHAPTER 3

1. R. H. Fletcher and K. M. Fairfield, "Vitamins for Chronic Disease Prevention in Adults: Clinical Applications," *JAMA*. 287 no. 23 (June 19, 2002): 3127–29.

2. J. Kliukiene et al., "Risk of Breast Cancer among Norwegian Women With Visual Impairment," *British Journal of Cancer* 84 (2001): 397–99.

3. J. Hansen, "Increased Breast Cancer Risk among Women Who Work Predominantly at Night," *Epidemiology* 12, no. 1 (2001): 74–77.

4. K. Doheny, "Can't Sleep? Adjust the Temperature," *WebMD*, March 2008, http://www.webmd.com/sleep-disorders/features/cant-sleep-adjust-the-temperature (accessed April 20, 2009).

5. Ibid.

6. U.S. Environmental Protection Agency, "About the Indoor Environments Division," http://epa.gov/iaq/aboutus.html (accessed April 20, 2009).

7. U.S. Environmental Protection Agency, "An Introduction to Indoor Air Quality: Volatile Organic Compounds (VOCs)," http://epa.gov/iaq/voc.html (accessed April 20, 2009).

8. J. Mulhall et al., "Importance of and Satisfaction with Sex among Men and Women Worldwide: Results of the Global Better Sex Survey," *Journal of Sexual Medicine* 5 (2008): 788–95.

THE BATHROOM: CHAPTER 4

1. A. Goodman, "Sources and Origins of Compounds of Emerging Concerns," *Proceedings of the Water Environment Federation, Compounds of Emerging Concern* (2007): 197–223, http://www.ingentaconnect.com/content/wef/wefproc/2007/00002007/00000006/art00017.

2. Environmental Working Group, "Body Burden: The Pollution in Newborns," http://ewg.org/reports/bodyburden2/execsumm.php (accessed February 20, 2010).

3. "Cosmetics: Product and Ingredient Safety," U.S. Food and Drug Administration, http://www.fda.gov/cosmetics/productandingredientsafety/default.htm (accessed July 1, 2010).

4. J. Nudelman et al., "Policy and Research Recommendations Emerging From the Scientific Evidence Connecting Environmental Factors and Breast Cancer," *International Journal of Occupational and Environmental Health* 15, no. 1 (2009): 79–101.

5. S. Epstein and R. Fitzgerald, *Toxic Beauty* (Dallas, TX: Benbella Books, 2009).

6. R. Sutton, "Adolescent Exposure to Cosmetic Chemicals of Concern," Environmental Working Group, http://www.ewg.org/reports/teens.2008 (accessed April 21, 2009).

7. Ibid.

8. V. Timm-Knudson et al., "Allergic Contact Dermatitis to Preservatives," *Dermatology Nursing* 18 (2006): 130–36.

9. U.S. Centers for Disease Control, Agency for Toxic Substances & Disease Registry, "Toxicological Profile for Aluminum: Health Effects," http://www.atsdr.cdc.gov/ToxProfiles/TP.asp?id=191&tid=34# (accessed February 20, 2010).

THE BATHROOM: CHAPTER 5

1. U.S. Centers for Disease Control, Agency for Toxic Substances & Disease Registry, "Toxicological Profile for Mercury: Health Effects," http://www.atsdr.cdc.gov/ToxProfiles/TP.asp?id=115&tid=24 (accessed February 20, 2010).

2. M. Wentz, *A Mouth Full of Poison*, (Rosarito Beach, Baja California: Medicis, 2004), 25-32.

3. Ibid., 4.

4. "Summary of Changes to the Classification of Dental Amalgam and Mercury," Food and Drug Administration, http://www.fda.gov/MedicalDevices/ProductsandMedicalProcedures/DentalProducts/DentalAmalgam/ucm171120.htm (accessed, April 25, 2010).

THE BATHROOM: CHAPTER 6

1. M. Mendoza, et al., "Pressure Rises to Stop Antibiotics in Agriculture," *Associated Press*, December 29, 2009.

2. A. E. Aiello et al., "Consumer Antibacterial Soaps: Effective or Just Risky?" *Clinical Infectious Diseases* 1, no. 45 (September 2007): S137–47.

3. L. Born, "Vaccinations: Parents' Informed Choice," Weston A Price Foundation (2005), http://www.westonaprice.org/children/vaccinations.html (accessed October 15, 2009).

4. Ibid.

5. M. D. Kogan, S. J. Blumberg, and L. A. Schieve, "Prevalence of Parent-Reported Diagnosis of Autism Spectrum Disorder Among Children in the US," *Pediatrics*, October 5, 2009.

6. A. Howd, "When Vaccines Do Harm to Kids," *American Gulf War Veterans Association* (2000), www.gulfwarvets.com/kids.htm (accessed October 15, 2009).

7. U. Erasmus, *Fats That Heal, Fats That Kill* (Burnaby BC, Canada: Alive Books, 1993).

8. "Cholesterol," Wikipedia, http://en.wikipedia.org/wiki/Cholesterol (accessed November 18, 2009).

9. Erasmus, *Fats That Heal, Fats That Kill.*

10. U. Ravnskov, "High Cholesterol May Protect Against Infections and Atherosclerosis," *QJM International Journal of Medicine* 96 (2003): 927–34.

11. "Mike's Calorie and Fat Gram Chart for 1000 Foods," http://www.caloriecountercharts.com/chart4a.htm (accessed June 10, 2010).

12. Erasmus, *Fats That Heal, Fats That Kill.*

13. "Small Diabetes Risk Is Not a Reason to Stop Taking Statins," *Medical News Today*, February 21, 2010, http://www.medicalnewstoday.com/articles/179779.php. (accessed February 26, 2010).

14. "Top 5 Lifestyle Changes to Reduce Cholesterol," Mayo Clinic, http//www.mayoclinic.com/health/reduce-cholesterol/CL00012 (accessed February 26, 2010).

15. J. O'Rourke, "Patients OD'ing on OTC Drugs: Warnings Not Sufficient, Some Contend," *Los Angeles Daily News*, December 23, 2006.

16. "Acetaminophen Side Effects," Online Lawyer Source, http://www. onlinelawyersource.com/acetaminophen/side-effects.html (accessed February 2, 2010).

17. R. Strand, *Death by Prescription: The Shocking Truth Behind an Overmedicated Nation* (Nashville, TN: Thomas Nelson, 2003).

18. Ibid., 208–09.

THE KITCHEN: CHAPTER 7

1. R. Strand, M.D. "*Healthy for Life* lecture series," 2009.

2. S. B. Eaton, M. J. Konner, and L. Cordain, "Diet-dependent Acid Load, Paleolithic Nutrition and Evolutionary Health Promotion," *American Journal of Clinical Nutrition* 91, no. 2 (February 2010): 295–97.

3. J. H. O'Keefe, Jr. and L. Cordain, "Cardiovascular Disease Resulting From a Diet and Lifestyle at Odds with Our Paleolithic Genome: How to Become a 21st-Century Hunter-Gatherer," *Mayo Clinic Proceedings* 79, no. 1 (January 2004): 101–08.

4. S. B. Eaton, "The Ancestral Human Diet: What Was It and Should It Be a Paradigm for Contemporary Nutrition?" *Proceedings of the Nutrition* Society 65 (2006): 1–6.

5. D. A. Bushinsky et al., "Proton-induced Physicochemical Calcium Release from Ceramic Apatite Disks," *Journal of Bone and Mineral Research* 9, no. 2 (February 1994): 213–20.

6. D. A. Bushinky et al., "Ion Microprobe Determination of Bone Surface Elements: Effects of Reduced Medium pH," *American Journal of Physiology* 250, no. 6 (June 1986): F1090–97; D. A. Bushinsky et al., "Physiochemical Effects of Acidosis on Bone Calcium Flux and Surface Ion Composition," *Journal of Bone and Mineral Research* 8, no. 1 (January 1993): 93–102; J. M. Chabala, R. Levi-Setti, and D. A. Bushinsky, "Alteration in Surface Ion Composition of Cultured Bone During Metabolic, But Not Respiratory, Acidosis," *American Journal of Physiology* 261, no. 1, pt. 2 (July 1991): F76–84.

7. D. A. Buchinsky et al., "Effects Of In Vivo Metabolic Acidosis on Midcortical Bone Ion Composition," *American Journal of Physiology* 277 (November 1999): F813–19.

8. D. A. Bushinsky, "Acid-base Imbalance and the Skeleton," *European Journal of Nutrition* 5, no. 40 (October 2001): 238–44.

9. M. Roland-Mieszkowski, "Cancer—A Biophysicist's Point of View," Digitalrecordings.com, July 21, 2004, http://www.digital-recordings.com/publ/cancer.html (accessed February 12, 2010).

10. J. A. Kellum, M. Song, and J. Li, "Science Review: Extracellular Acidosis and the Immune Response: Clinical and Physiological Implications," *Critical Care* 8, no. 5 (October 2005): 331–36.

11. M. Huang et al., "Non-small Cell Lung Cancer Cyclooxygenase-2-Dependant Regulation of Cytokine Balance in Lymphocytes and Macrophages: Up-regulation of Interleukin 10 and Down-regulation of Interleukin 12 Production," *Cancer Research* 58, no. 6 (March 1998): 1208–16; C. N. Baxevanis et al., "Elevated Prostaglandin E2 Production by Monocytes Is Responsible For the Depressed Levels of Natural Killer and Lumphokine-activated Killer Cell Function in Patients With Breast Cancer," *Cancer* 72, no. 2 (July 1993): 491–501.

12. J. M. Wallace, "Nutritional and Botanical Modulation of the Inflammatory Cascade—Eicosanoids, Cyclooxygenases, and Lipoxygenases—As an Adjunct in Cancer Therapy," *Integrated Cancer Therapy* 1, no. 1 (March 2002): 7–37; A. B. Crumley et al., "Evaluation of an Inflammation-Based Prognostic Score in Patients with Inoperable Gastrooesophageal Cancer," *British Journal of Cancer* 94, no. 5 (March 2006): 637–41; A. M. Al Murri et al., "Evaluation of an Inflammation-based Prognostic Score (GPS) in Patients with Metastatic Breast Cancer," *British Journal of Cancer* 94, no. 2 (January 2006): 227–30.

13. J. Challem, "The pH Nutrition Guide to Acid/Alkaline Balance," Natural News, 2010, http://www.naturalnews.com/report_acid_alkaline_pH_1.html (accessed February 10, 2010).

14. L. A. Frassetto et al., "Adverse Effects of Sodium Chloride on Bone in the Aging Human Population Resulting from Habitual Consumption of Typical American Diets," *Journal of Nutrition* 138, no. 2 (February 2008): 419S–22S; P. Frings-Meuthen, N. Baecker, and M. Heer, "Low-grade Metabolic Acidosis May Be the Cause of Sodium Chloride-induced Exaggerated Bone Resorption," *Journal of Bone Mineral Research* 23, no. 4 (April 2008): 517–24.

THE KITCHEN: CHAPTER 8

1. L. Song and P. J. Thornalley, "Effect of Storage, Processing, and Cooking on Glucosinolate Content of Brassica Vegetables," *Food Chem Toxicol* 2, no. 45 (February 2007): 216–24; G. F. Yuan et al., "Effects of Different Cooking Methods on Health-promoting Compounds of Broccoli," *Journal of Zhejiang*

University, Science B 8, no. 10 (August 2009): 580–88; V. Rungapamestry et al., "Changes in Glucosinolate Concentrations, Myrosinase Activity, and Production of Metabolites of Glucosinolates in Cabbage," *Journal of Agricultural Food Chemistry* 4, no. 54 (October 2006): 7628–34.

2. A. M. Jimenez-Monreal et al., "Influence of Cooking Methods on Antioxidant Activity of Vegetables," *Journal of Food Science* 74, no.3 (April 2009): H97–103.

3. H. A. Schroeder, "Losses of Vitamins and Trace Minerals Resulting from Processing and Preservation of Foods," *American Journal of Clinical Nutrition* 24, no. 5 (May 1971): 562–73.

4. D. J. McKillop et al., "The Effect of Different Cooking Methods on Folate Retention in Various Foods that Are amongst the Major Contributors to Folate Intake in the UK Diet," *British Journal of Nutrition* 6, no. 88 (December 2002): 681–88.

5. L. Song and P. J. Thornalley, "Effect of Storage, Processing, and Cooking on Glucosinolate Content of Brassica Vegetables," *Food Chemistry and Toxicology* 45, no. 2 (February 2007): 216–24.

6. M. Kimura and Y. Itokawa, "Cooking Losses of Minerals in Foods and Its Nutritional Significance," *Journal of Nutritional Science and Vitaminology* 36 (1990): S25–32.

7. "Microwave Ovens and Food Safety," *Health Canada,* July 2005, http://www.hc-sc.gc.ca/hl-vs/iyh-vsv/prod/micro-f-a-eng.php (accessed Oct. 1, 2009).

8. "Heterocyclic amines in cooked meats," National Cancer Institute, September 15, 2004, http://www.cancer.gov/cancertopics/factsheet/Risk/heterocyclic-amines (accessed April 21, 2010)

9. "High-temperature Cooking and the World's Healthiest Foods," George Mateljan Foundation, http://www.whfoods.com/genpage.php?tname=george&dbid=122 (accessed April 21, 2010).

10. F. Mangano, "The Hidden Health Hazards of Grilling and Barbecuing," http://ezinearticles.com/?The-Hidden-Health-Hazards-of-Grilling-And-Barbecuing&id=243933 (accessed April 21, 2010).

11. J. Houlihan et al., "Canaries in the Kitchen: Teflon Toxicosis," Environmental Working Group, May 2003, http://www.ewg.org/reports/toxicteflon (accessed February 19, 2010).

12. Ibid.

13. Ibid.

14. "Important Cooking Safety Tips," Dupont, http://www2.dupont.com/Teflon/en_US/assets/downloads/cooking_safely/safety_tips.pdf (accessed February 22, 2010).

15. "A Pictorial Walk Through the 20th Century," U.S. Department of Labor, http://www.msha.gov/century/canary/canary.asp (accessed February 22, 2010).

16. "Styrene," Environmental Protection Agency, January 2000, http://www.epa.gov/ttn/atw/hlthef/styrene.html#ref5 (accessed March 5, 2010).

17. L. Castle, M. Kelly, and J. Gilbert, "Migration of Mineral Hydrocarbons into Foods" and "Polystyrene, ABS, and Waxed Paperboard Containers for Dairy Products," *Food Additives and Contaminants* 10, no. 2 (March 1993): 167–74; M. Kempf, "Occurrence of 2,2,4Trimethyl-1,3-Pentanediol Monoisobutyrate (Texanol) in Foods Packed in Polystyrene and Polypropylene Cups," *Food Additives and Contaminants Part A Chemistry Analysis Control, Exposure and Risk Assessment* 26, no. 4 (April 2009): 563–67; P. G. Murphy, D. A. MacDonald, and T. D. Lickly, "Styrene Migration from General-purpose and High-impact Polystyrene into Food-simulating Solvents," *Food and Chemical Toxicology* 30, no. 3 (March 1992): 225–32; M. S. Tawfik and A. Huyghebaert, "Polystyrene Cups and Containers: Styrene Migration," *Food Additives and Contamination* 15, no. 5 (July 1998): 592–99; W. J. Uhde and H. Woggon, "New Results on Migration Behavior of Benzophenone-based UV Absorbents from Polyolefins in Foods," *Nahrung* 20, no. 2 (1976): 185–94; O. Vitrac et al., "Contamination of Packaged Food by Substances Migrating from a Direct-contact Plastic Layer: Assessment Using a Generic Quantitative Household Scale Methodology," *Food Additives and Contamination* 24, no. 1 (January 2007): 75–94; W. J. Uhde and H. Woggon, "Antistatic Finishing of Plastics from Food Hygiene and Toxicological Viewpoints," *Nahrung* 21, no. 3 (1977): 235–45.

18. J. E. Matiella and T. C. Hsieh, "Volatile Compounds in Scrambled Eggs," *Journal of Food Science* 56, no. 2 (March 1991): 387–90.

19. P. Alonso-Magdalena, "The Estrogenic Effect of Bisphenol A Disrupts Pancreatic Beta-cell Function in Vivo and Induces Insulin Resistance," *Environmental Health Perspectives* 114, no. 1 (January 2006): 106–12; P. Goettlich, "Get Plastic Out of Your Diet," Mindfully.org, November 16, 2003, http://www.mindfully.org/Plastic/Plasticizers/Out-Of-Diet-PG5nov03.htm (accessed December 10, 2009).

20. G. Latini, "Peroxisome Proliferator-activated Receptors as Mediators of Phthalate-induced Effects in the Male and Female Reproductive Tract:

Epidemiological and Experimental Evidence," PPAR Research, 2008 (accession number 359267) (accessed July 1, 2010); J. D. Meeker, A. M. Calafat, and R. Hauser, "Urinary Metabolites of Di(2-ethylhexyl) Phthalate Are Associated with Decreased Steroid Hormone Levels in Adult Men," *Journal of Andrology* 30, no. 3 (May 2009): 287–97; J. D. Meeker, S. Sathyanarayana, and S. H. Swan, "Phthalates and Other Additives in Plastics: Human Exposure and Associated Health Outcomes," *Philosophical Transactions of the Royal Society of London Biological Sciences* 364, no. 1526 (July 2009): 2097–113; N. Pant et al., "Correlation of Phthalate Exposures with Semen Quality," *Toxicology and Applied Pharmacology* 231, no. 1 (August 2008): 112–16; K. P. Phillips and N. Tanphaichitr, "Human Exposure to Endocrine Disrupters and Semen Quality," *Journal of Toxicology and Environmental Health B Critical Review* 11, no. 3–4 (March 2008): 188–220; H. E. Virtanen, "Testicular Dysgenesis Syndrome and the Development and Occurrence of Male Reproductive Disorders," *Toxicology and Applied Pharmacology* 1, no. 207 (September 2005): 501–05; J. J. Wirth et al. "A Pilot Study Associating Urinary Concentrations of Phthalate Metabolites and Semen Quality," *Systems Biology in Reproductive Medicine* 54, no. 3 (May 2008): 143–54.

21. "Plastic Containers Buying Guide," National Geographic, http://www.thegreenguide.com/buying-guide/plastic-containers (accessed March 5, 2010).

22. K. R. Weiss, "Plague of Plastic Chokes the Seas," *Los Angeles Times*, August 2, 2006, http://www.latimes.com/news/printedition/la-me-ocean2aug02,0,5594900.story (accessed July 1, 2010).

THE KITCHEN: CHAPTER 9

1. K. J. Duffey and B. M. Popkin, "Shifts in Patterns and Consumption of Beverages Between 1965 and 2002," *Obesity* 15 (2007): 2739–47, http://www.nature.com/oby/journal/v15/n11/full/oby2007326a.html (accessed July 2, 2010).

2. C. Duhigg, "Millions in U.S. Drink Dirty Water, Records Show," *New York Times*, December 7, 2009.

3. Ibid.

4. "Fluoride in Drinking Water: A Scientific Review of EPA's Standards," *National Research Council*, March 22, 2006.

5. Ibid.

6. "Fluoride and Infant Formula: Frequently Asked Questions," American Dental Association, http://www.ada.org/4052.aspx (accessed March 15, 2010).

7. E. D. Olsen, "Bottled Water: Pure Drink or Pure Hype?" Natural Resources Defense Council, February 1999, http://www.nrdc.org/water/drinking/bw/bwinx.asp and http://www.nrdc.org/water/drinking/qbw.asp (accessed July 1, 2010).

8. "Calcium and Milk: What's Best for Your Bones and Health?" Harvard School of Public Health, www.hsph.harvard.edu/ . . . /what-should . . . /calcium-full-story/ (accessed January 9, 2010).

9. B. Avery et al., "Lowering Dietary Protein to U.S. Recommended Dietary Allowance Levels Reduces Urinary Calcium Excretion and Bone Resorption in Young Women," *Journal of Clinical Endocrinology & Metabolism* (accession number 89:3801–07. 2004).

10. S. Brown, *Better Bones, Better Body* (Los Angeles: Keats Publishing, 2000), 81–114.

11. "Calcium and Milk: What's Best for Your Bones and Health?"

12. C. S. Johnston, D. L. Bowling, "Stability of Ascorbic Acid in Commercially Available Orange Juices," *Journal of the American Dietetic Association* 102, no. 4 (2002): 525–29.

LIVING AREAS: CHAPTER 10

1. U.S. Environmental Protection Agency, "An Introduction to Indoor Air Quality: Volatile Organic Compounds (VOCs)," http://epa.gov/iaq/voc.html (accessed April 20, 2009).

2. A. C. Bronstein et al., "2008 Annual Report of the American Association of Poison Control Centers' National Poison Data System, (NPDS) 26th Annual Report," *Clinical Toxicology* 47(2009): 911–1084.

3. "A Little about Baking Soda," *Baking Soda Book*, http://www.bakingsodabook.co.uk/baking_soda_book_a_little_about_baking_soda.shtml (accessed April 4, 2010).

4. "Ten Uses for Borax," Essortment, http://www.essortment.com/home/usesforborax_swox.htm (accessed April 4, 2010).

5. "Using Essential Oils to Clean and Disinfect," Housekeeping Matters, http://housekeepingmatters.com/using-essential-oils-to-clean-and-disinfect/ (accessed April 4, 2010).

LIVING AREAS: CHAPTER 11

1. S. Kovach, "The Hidden Dangers of Cell Phone Radiation," *Life Extension Magazine*, August 2009, http://www.lef.org/magazine/mag2007/aug2007_report_cellphone_radiation_01.htm (accessed May 10, 2010).

2. "Cell Phone Radiofrequency Radiation Studies," National Toxicology Program, http://www.niehs.nih.gov/health/docs/cell-phone-fact-sheet.pdf (accessed October 4, 2009).

3. "Mobile Telephones and Health Effects," Australian Radiation Protection and Nuclear Safety Agency, 2009, http://www.arpansa.gov.au/mobilephones/index.cfm (accessed October 6, 2009).

4. L. Hardell and M. Carlberg, "Mobile Phones, Cordless Phones, and the Risk for Brain Tumors," *International Journal of Oncology* 35 (2009): 5–17.

5. H. Divan et al., "Prenatal and Postnatal Exposure to Cell Phone Use and Behavioral Problems in Children," *Epidemiology* 19 (2008): 523–29.

6. "Worldwide PC Adoption Forecast, 2007 to 2015," Forrester, June 11, 2007, http://www.forrester.com/rb/Research/worldwide_pc_adoption_forecast%2C_2007_to_2015/q/id/42496/t/2 (accessed May 3, 2010).

7. T. Liu and M. N. Potenza, "Problematic Internet Use: Clinical Implications," *CNS Spectrums* 12, no. 6 (2007): 453–66; B. Dell'Osso et al., "Epidemiologic and Clinical Updates On Impulse Control Disorders; A Critical Review," *European Archives of Psychiatry and Clinical Neuroscience* 256 (2006): 464–75.

8. J. J. Block, "Pathological Computer Use In the USA," 2007 International Symposium on the Counseling and Treatment of Youth Internet Addiction, Seoul, Korea, National Youth Commission (2007): 433; K. W. Beard and E. M. Wolf, "Modification in the Proposed Diagnostic Criteria for Internet Addiction," *Cyberpsychol Behaviour* 4 (2001): 377–83; R. Pies, "Should DSM-V Designate 'Internet Addiction' a Mental Disorder?" *Psychiatry* 6, no. 2 (2009): 31–37.

9. Liu and Potenza, "Problematic Internet Use."

10. K. S. Young, "Internet Addiction: The Emergence of a New Clinical Disorder," *Cyberpsychological Behaviour* 11 (1998): 237–44.

THE GARAGE AND YARD: CHAPTER 12

1. A. Schlapia and S. S. Morris, "Architectural, Behavioral and Environmental Factors Associated with VOCs in Anchorage Homes," Anchorage Air Pollution

Control Agency, 1996, http://www.muni.org/Departments/health/environment/
AirQ/Pages/AirQualitySpecialStudies.aspx (accessed July 1, 2010); S. J.
Emmerich, J. E. Gorfain, and C. Howard-Reed, "Air and Pollutant Transport
from Attached Garages to Residential Living Spaces—Literature Review and
Field Tests," *International Journal of Ventilation* 2, no. 3, http://fire.nist.gov/
bfrlpubs/build03/PDF/b03067.pdf (accessed July 1, 2010).

THE GARAGE AND YARD: CHAPTER 13

1. F. D. Roosevelt, "Letter to All State Governors on a Uniform Soil Conservation
    Law," February 26, 1937.

2. T. Takano et al., "Urban Residential Environments and Senior Citizens'
    Longevity in Megacity Areas: The Importance of Walkable Green Spaces," *Journal
    of Epidemiology and Community Health* 56 (December 2002): 913–18.

3. G. T. Miller, *Sustaining the Earth* (Pacific Grove, CA: Thompson Learning, Inc.,
    2004), 211–16.

4. "Antarctic Melt Releasing DDT, Tainting Penguins," National Geographic News,
    May 12, 2008, http://news.nationalgeographic.com/news/2008/05/080512-
    penguins-ddt.html (accessed June 29, 2010).

5. "Chlordane," Eco-USA Toxic Chemicals, http://www.eco-usa.net/toxics/
    chemicals/chlordane.shtml (accessed June 29, 2010).

6. R. Lewis et al., "Measuring and Reducing Exposure to the Pollutants in House
    Dust," *American Journal of Public Health* 85 (1995): 1168.

7. R. Renner, "Curse This House," *New Scientist*, iss. 2289, May 5, 2001.

8. U.S. Environmental Protection Agency, "Pesticides and Food: Health Problems
    Pesticides May Pose," http://www.epa.gov/pesticides/food/risks.htm (accessed
    June 10, 2010).

9. Center for Sustainable Systems, University of Michigan, 2009, "U.S.
    Environmental Footprint Factsheet," Pub. no. CSS08–08, http://css.snre.umich.
    edu/css_doc/CSS08–08.pdf (accessed July 1, 2010).

10. W. D. Schmidt et al., "Effects of Long Versus Short Bout Exercise on Fitness and
    Weight Loss in Overweight Females," *Journal of the American College of Nutrition*
    20 (2001): 494–501.

11. A. R. Ness et al., "Objectively Measured Physical Activity and Fat Mass in a Large Cohort of Children," *PLOS Medicine* 4, no. 3 (2007): e97, http://www.plosmedicine.org/article/info%3Adoi%2F10.1371%2Fjournal.pmed.0040097 (accessed July 1, 2010).

EPILOGUE TWO

1. A. McGinn, "Phasing Out Persistent Organic Pollutants," in *State of the World*, ed. Worldwatch Institute, chap. 5, 79–100 (New York: Norton, 2000).

2. Environmental Defense Fund, "Toxic Ignorance: The Continuing Absence of Basic Health Testing for Top-selling Chemicals in the United States," in *The Current State of Ignorance About Chemical Hazards*, chap. 2, 11–15 (1997), http://www.edf.org/documents/243_toxicignorance.pdf (accessed May 28, 2010).

Index

sleep's role in repair of, 56–57

CFLs (Compact Fluorescent Lights), 182–183

Change
    improving personal environments, 248–250
    participating in, 244–245

Chemicals
    absorption through skin, 69, 225
    added to personal-care products, 66–67, 70–71
    aluminum, 81–85
    dry cleaning, 29–30
    effects of preservatives on cells, 73
    flame retardants, 23, 37–38
    fluorine/fluoride, 164–165
    formaldehyde, 76–77
    found in aerosols, 79–80
    hazards of household cleaners, 183–189
    HFRs, 23
    makeup of plastics, 156–157
    mattresses treated with, 37–39
    overexposure to, 248–250
    parabens, 74–76
    PFCs, 23
    PVC, 22
    sensing with nose, 18, 186
    synthetic clothing and, 22–23
    treating drinking water, 162
    used in plastics, 149–151
    VOCs, 26–27, 30, 52–53, 182, 188
    See also specific chemicals

Children
    adding fluoride to water, 163–165
    dangers of fluoride toothpaste for, 87–88
    dirt's effect on, 7, 179

effect of EMFs on, 45
    hazards of cell phones for, 202–204
    limiting use of electrical devices, 209
    mercury fillings for, 93
    monitoring Internet use, 208
    parabens and sexual development of, 74–76
    sensitivity to artificial fragrances, 26
    susceptibility to toxins, 186–187
    vaccines for, 102–106
    vulnerability to pesticides, 232
    See also Infants

Children's Hunger Fund (CHF), 8

Chlordane, 231

Chlorine gas, 188

Cholesterol, 106–110
    about, 106–107
    body's need for, 108–109, 111
    lifestyle solutions lowering, 111
    protecting, 109–110
    statins for, 111

Clean Air Act, 53

Cleaning, 180–197
    changing habits of, 209–210
    dangers of household cleaners, 187–189
    dry cleaning clothes, 29–33
    greener cleaners, 190–193
    homemade solutions for, 194
    living areas, 183–187
    pollutants in living areas, 181–182
    quiz on, 180
    selecting vacuums for, 196
    steam cleaners, 195–196
    sunshine and ventilation for, 192–193

Clothing
    alternatives for dry cleaning, 31–32

effects of Internet addiction,
207–209

electrical devices in, 198–209

evaluating health of, 177–179

healthy cleaning solutions, 183–187

pesticides migrating into, 231–233

pollutants in, 181–182

removing shoes before entering,
195, 221–222, 231–232

repainting, 182

solutions for, 209–211

testing for contaminants, 196–197

vacuums for, 196

Lymphatic fluid, 33–34, 37

Mad Hatter, 90–91

Magnesium, 48, 88

Maintaining bodily balance, 130

Marketing campaigns
food, 124–125
home cleansers, 185
merchandising cleanliness, 25–29

Mattresses, 37–39

Maximum safe levels of toxins, 71–72

Meat, 99–100, 145–146

Melatonin, 19, 49–50, 56

Men
clothing for, 35–37
phthalates and effects on, 154

Mercury
detoxing, 94–95
found in vaccines, 103
toxicity of fillings with, 89–95
vaccines preserved with, 103–104

Microwaves
avoiding EMFs of, 145
effect on plasticware, 151
preparing food with, 143–145

technology for, 45

Milk, 169–171

Minerals
acid load and, 132
aluminium and deficiency in, 84
calcium, 44, 45, 170–171
effect on cell repair, 48
needed for healthy teeth, 88
reducing oxidative stress, 110

Mold, 195, 196

Moms against Mercury, 93

Mouth Full of Poison, A (Wentz), 95

Mouthwashes, 88–89

Mudrooms, 222

N-acetyl L-cysteine, 94

National Academy of Science, 26

National Geographic "Green Guide," 155

National Research Council, 163

Natural alternatives. *See* Greening
environments

Nature
exercising outdoors, 239–241
healing properties of, 227–229
See also Yard

Net acid load, 132–133

New York Times, 162

No-iron fabrics, 23, 24

Nonspray personal products, 79

Nose
airing out homes, 181–182,
192–193
detecting toxicity with, 5, 18,
25–29, 186
inhaling cleanser smells, 189
sensitivities to bedroom air
pollution, 52–55
testing dry-cleaned clothes, 31

THE HEALTHY HOME

Ready to Get Started?

Use your personal pass to myhealthyhome.com

Enter the unique access code below on myhealthyhome.com to unlock free, exclusive content, including:

- A Healthy Home assessment that you can save and update as you make progress
- MORE Simple Solutions to improve your Healthy Home score
- Further resources on the subjects discussed in *The Healthy Home*
- The latest news on health issues that could affect your family
- Select discounts for healthier products from trusted vendors

Log on to myhealthyhome.com today to begin taking simple steps toward a healthier home for you and your family.

Unique Web Access Code
5DWK3A1HH

myhealthyhome.com